Traumatic Brain Injury - Recent Advances and Challenges

Edited by Ioannis Mavroudis and Alin Ciobica

Published in London, United Kingdom

Traumatic Brain Injury - Recent Advances and Challenges
http://dx.doi.org/10.5772/intechopen.110973
Edited by Ioannis Mavroudis and Alin Ciobica

Contributors
Abdel Karim Qudah, Ahmad Tamimi, Alin Ciobica, Ashani Couchman, Faleh Tamimi, Fatima Zahra Kamal, Foivos Petridis, Fuxiang Zhu, Hanqiang Shi, Ioannis Mavroudis, Iskandar Tamimi, Jiayuan Zhai, Leighton J. Reynolds, Leslie Griffin, Lie Xiong, Lifeng Qian, Madeleine Bain, Manuela Padurariu, Mohamad Barbarawi, Motari Omariba, Pauline N. Kariuki, Sunfeng Pan, Thomas Milton, Wanchao Yang, Yanbing Feng, Yanbo Shi, Zeynep Karakuzu Güngör, Zhongwei Yu

First published in London, United Kingdom, 2025 by IntechOpen
IntechOpen is the global imprint of INTECHOPEN LIMITED, registered in England and Wales, registration number: 11086078, 167-169 Great Portland Street, London, W1W 5PF, United Kingdom

For EU product safety concerns: IN TECH d.o.o., Prolaz Marije Krucifikse Kozulić 3, 51000 Rijeka, Croatia, info@intechopen.com or visit our website at intechopen.com.

British Library Cataloguing-in-Publication Data
A catalogue record for this book is available from the British Library

Traumatic Brain Injury - Recent Advances and Challenges
Edited by Ioannis Mavroudis and Alin Ciobica
p. cm.
Print ISBN 978-0-85466-944-8
Online ISBN 978-0-85466-943-1
eBook (PDF) ISBN 978-0-85466-945-5

Meet the editors

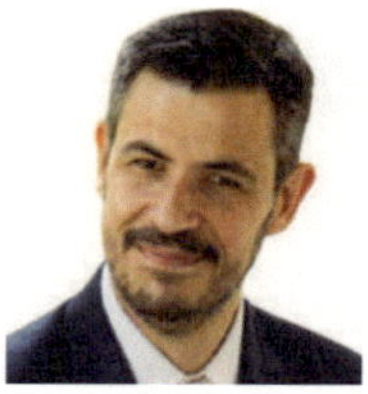

Dr. Ioannis Mavroudis is a consultant neurologist and Senior Lecturer with a special interest in mild traumatic brain injury (mTBI) and neurodegeneration. He holds a Ph.D. in neuropathology and neuromorphology and has been actively involved in research since 2005. Dr. Mavroudis has published over 80 peer-reviewed papers and authored more than eight books in the fields of neurology and neuroscience. With extensive clinical experience, he has worked in traumatic brain injury and has led recovery planning for mTBI patients. He has taught neuroanatomy and neuropathology in Greece, clinical neurology as a visiting assistant professor at the University of Cyprus, and served as a visiting lecturer at the University of Leeds. Recently, he was elected Assistant Professor of Neurology at Aristotle University of Thessaloniki. Dr. Mavroudis is also a leader in medicolegal neurology, providing expert opinions on concussion cases and directing efforts to improve early screening and rehabilitation for head injuries. His work integrates cutting-edge research with practical applications in concussion diagnosis, monitoring, and treatment. As the academic editor of this book, he brings his expertise in both clinical and research aspects of concussions, offering a comprehensive perspective on the subject.

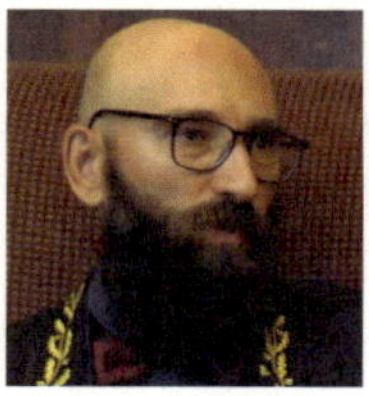

Dr. Alin Ciobica has over 20 years of research experience in studying various behavioral tests and animal models of neuropsychiatric disorders, as well as the relevance of oxidative stress status in this context.

Contents

Preface

Traumatic Brain Injuries (TBI) represent a significant and growing concern in modern medicine, affecting individuals across all age groups and professions, from athletes and military personnel to the general population. Mild traumatic brain injury (mTBI) can have lasting effects on cognitive function, emotional well-being, and overall quality of life. As our understanding of the pathophysiology, diagnosis, and management of TBI advances, this volume brings together leading experts to present a comprehensive overview of the latest developments in the field.

This book explores fundamental and emerging aspects of TBI research, covering key areas such as the biomechanics of brain injury, advancements in neuroimaging, biomarkers for diagnosis, and evidence-based rehabilitation strategies. We delve into the clinical presentation of TBI, discussing the acute and chronic consequences of head trauma and the importance of early and accurate diagnosis. Special emphasis is placed on objective assessment tools, including neurocognitive testing and eye-tracking technologies, which enhance diagnostic precision and treatment monitoring. Furthermore, this volume addresses the complex intersection of TBIs with neurodegenerative diseases, post-traumatic stress disorder, and functional neurological disorders, highlighting the long-term implications of repeated head injuries.

The book also provides insights into the medicolegal aspects of TBI, including forensic evaluations, return-to-play protocols in sports, and disability assessments in occupational settings. By integrating perspectives from neurology, sports medicine, neuropsychology, and rehabilitation sciences, this volume serves as a vital resource for clinicians, researchers, and policymakers seeking to enhance patient care and public health outcomes.

I extend my deepest gratitude to the contributing authors for their expertise and dedication in advancing the science of TBIs. I also wish to thank the editorial team for their invaluable assistance in compiling this volume. Finally, I am grateful to my colleagues and mentors who have shaped my understanding of traumatic brain injury and its broader implications.

Dr. Ioannis Mavroudis MD, PhD, FRCP
Consultant Neurologist,
Department of Neuroscience,
Leeds Teaching Hospitals,
NHS Trust,
Leeds, UK

Honorary Senior Lecturer,
Leeds University,
Leeds, UK

Assistant Professor of Neurology,
Aristotle University of Thessaloniki,
Thessaloniki, Greece

Dr. Alin Ciobica
Department of Biology,
Faculty of Biology,
Alexandru Ioan Cuza University,
Iasi, Romania

Centre of Biomedical Research,
Romanian Academy,
Iasi, Romania

Academy of Romanian Scientists,
Bucharest, Romania

Preclinical Department,
Apollonia University,
Iasi, Romania

Section 1

Introduction to Traumatic Brain Injury (TBI)

Chapter 1

Perspective Chapter: A Case Presentation – The Progression of an Unrecognized Traumatic Brain Injury from Childhood to Young Adulthood

Leighton J. Reynolds

Abstract

This chapter explores how a concussion sustained during childhood becomes a neurodegenerative disease process in the brain, first manifesting symptoms during adolescence. The patient (Mr. A), a 21-year-old college student, initially presented with serious issues related to cognitive decline. These issues had forced him to drop out of college because he could not focus effectively during his classes. Cognitive decline is one of the four baskets of symptoms used to diagnose concussion and post-concussion syndrome symptoms. The other three baskets of symptoms include physical symptoms, social and emotional issues, and sleep disturbances. The author tracks this case using a model developed for understanding and working with traumatic brain injury (TBI) patients: the four interlocking architectures the brain develops in response to being traumatized. They are: ARCHITECTURE ONE: A Shock Trauma/Traumatic Shock. ARCHITECTURE TWO: Electrical and Chemical Imbalances in the Brain. ARCHITECTURE THREE: Disrupting Homeostatic Balance and the Development of Allostatic Load. ARCHITECTURE FOUR: The Perfect Storm in the Brain. This chapter will focus on the symptomatology of Architecture Two: what is happening with the brain/mind during this architecture, how this is manifested in the patient's behavior, and how to treat a brain injury at this stage of the interlocking architectures. Architectures here refer to the brain's response to being traumatized and its attempts to reorganize itself. This model can also be applied to other injuries to the brain including strokes, seizures, transient ischemic attacks, infections, and autoimmune responses in the brain.

Keywords: traumatic brain injury, concussions, post-concussion syndrome, brain/mind, neuro-psychoanalysis, four baskets of symptoms

1. Introduction

A 21-year-old college student (Mr. A) was referred with the presentation: "I'm confused all the time, and I have no idea why?" At the time he began treatment with, no one had ever mentioned that he might be suffering from post-concussion syndrome (PCS). He had suffered an obvious concussion at age 8, and there were several probable concussions after that. However, up until adolescence, his development appeared to be normal, so everyone assumed he was just fine. The original concussion had occurred when he slipped off a picnic bench and struck his head on concrete, causing him to black out. He had minor complaints when his parents brought him to the ER (nausea and vomiting), but after an MRI, which showed nothing significant, he was sent home with his parents. Everything appeared normal following this incident and for years afterward. The idea that he had, or could have had, post-concussion syndrome, was nowhere on anyone's medical radar.

When Mr. A hit adolescence (ages 14, 15, 16), he began to struggle with a host of "weird issues" that he kept mostly to himself. By this time in his life, he was on his way to becoming a third-degree black belt in Karate, so what could have been going wrong? But listening to him in my office at age 21, I understood the symptomatology he described as falling into the category of cognitive decline, one of the four baskets of symptoms that occur following a concussion. The other three are physical symptoms, social and emotional issues, and sleep disturbances.

What exactly was he having difficulty with? He listed the following as his "new normal," which he believed began when he was a sophomore in high school:

Blurred vision (that made it difficult for him to focus on anything, especially when he was stressed).

Chronic fatigue (which was a constant struggle for him).

Increased sensitivity to light and sound (especially when he as around bright lights).

Increased inflammation in his body (although he was not exactly sure how he knew this). His motto was: above all do not complain about anything.

During his college classes he had difficulty focusing. And this was causing him a lot of problems because he could not track the lectures, and he could not follow through with his homework.

He noticed that his memory was a problem (especially his short-term memory).

He noticed that his brain was easily overwhelmed (and that it would shut down under these circumstances).

Several years before he began working with me, he had a serious meltdown during which he was hallucinating, felt he was going off the deep end, and then abruptly withdrew from the university and returned home.

He was aware that he had experiences of depersonalization (during which he did not know that he was a real person) and derealization (during which he did not feel that his surroundings were real).

He was taking Strattera (an anti-psychotic medicine) for a while (which helped him focus and do better in school, but it tended to magnify his emotional states, making them very difficult to manage, and he stopped the medication).

Hence, his major complaint when he began treatment with me: "I do not know how to understand why I am so confused all the time and everything I do is a struggle."

How do we understand the above symptomatology, which is very wide-ranging and identical to the symptomatology of post-concussion syndrome? And could any of his presenting symptoms have anything to do with the concussion he sustained at age 8? Over the past 7 years (working with traumatic brain injury patients), I have developed a model for understanding the progression of a traumatic brain injury. In my experience, all serious trauma to the head creates a neurodegenerative disease process in the brain/mind, especially if not treated immediately. It is progressive across four

DOI: http://dx.doi.org/10.5772/intechopen.1004377

interlocking phases as the brain/mind works to adjust to being traumatized. I describe these interlocking phases as architectures the brain/mind constructs in response to being traumatized in "The Complex Architecture and Healing of Traumatic Brain Injuries: Listening To The Brain" (Cambridge Scholars Press, August 2023). The four architectures are:

- ARCHITECTURE ONE: Shock Trauma/Traumatic Shock[1].
- ARCHITECTURE TWO: Electrical and Chemical Imbalances in the Brain.
- ARCHITECTURE THREE: Disrupting Homeostatic Balance and the Development of Allostatic Load[2].
- ARCHITECTURE FOUR: The Perfect Storm in the Brain.

And my answer to the question is yes! The effects of one concussion and post-concussion syndrome can last years, especially if unrecognized and untreated. This case is an example of what I see all too often in my office, the long-term effects of concussion and post-concussion syndrome. All too often, this symptomatology goes unrecognized and hence untreated. In this chapter, I explore how Architecture Two is played out in the life of this patient. The question here is: What do electrical and chemical breakdowns in the brain have to do with the symptoms my patient is experiencing?

2. Dialog

Let us begin with the patient.

P. "Dr. Reynolds, I think this is my new, new normal!"

Dr. R. "And how would you describe this new, new normal for you?"

P. "I'm not saying that I like this, but here goes."

P. "I'm actually depressed and anxious all the time."

P. "I do realize that I dissociate a lot, especially when I'm under a lot of stress."

P. "I get lost a lot going from one place to another."

P. "It's easy for me to get overstimulated."

P. "I am aware of the fact that I do not absorb and process information very well."

P. "I often feel that I am just walking around in a dream state, just like I was dreaming."

P. "I'm always trying to keep face, and not let anyone see how much I'm suffering."

P. "Depending on what I define as my element, I get very anxious when I know that I'm not in control of things."

P. "I am sadly aware that I cannot keep up with the pace of life."

P. "I'm always in fear of the unknown."

Dr. R. "Any ideas of what would help you in the face of the unknown to you?"

---

[1] For a further description of Architectures One, Two Three, and Four see "The Complex Architecture and Healing of Traumatic Brain Injuries," from Cambridge Scholars Publishing, August 2023.

[2] For a further detailed presentation of Architecture One see: "Listening To The Brain/Recovering The Brain," at SOJ Medical and Clinical Case Reports (23-CR-524) from Stephypublishers.group (2023).

P. "Well...I can think of 3 things: (1) Reduce the demands on my brain as you have suggested. (2) Pre-plan things so there are fewer unknowns and uncertainties. (3) Make sure that I'm in control of my surroundings."

Fortunately for my patient, he was able to follow through on his own suggestions and thus begin his healing process (his healing ecology).

3. The brain injury

If these are examples of Mr. A.'s behavior and what he struggles with, what exactly is going on in his brain/mind?

Moving from the Behavior to the Biology:

We know that a traumatic brain injury can lead to a range of pathophysiological changes that are serious and very wide ranging. Including:

- Dysregulated cerebral blood flow.
- Impaired cerebral oxygenation.
- Glutamate excitotoxicity (see below for an explanation).
- Blood-brain Barrier.
- Cerebral edema (swelling in the brain).
- Oxidative and nitrative (nitrosative) stress (see below).
- Cerebral inflammation.
- Hypo and hyper-perfusion (see below).
- Mitochondrial dysfunction.
- Hemorrhage.
- Hyperemia (blood vessels are filled with more blood than usual).

I understand the above physiological problems as evidence that normal brain function has been disrupted. Further over time, disruptions in brain/mind functioning lead to a breakdown in brain/mind functioning. This is what my patient was dealing with when he began treatment: the transition from brain/mind dysfunction to a brain/mind breakdown as the disease process of neurodegeneration continues on its downward, cascading course. These are the dynamics of Architecture Two as the brain/mind is working to readjust itself to being traumatized. But not doing it very well.

Let us look at several of these troubling areas exploring the arena of neurodegeneration, which I believe is causing my patients difficult symptoms.

Oxidative stress is caused by an imbalance of free radicals and antioxidants in the brain that leads to cell and tissue damage and death. Normally, cells will produce free radicals as a part of the normal metabolic process. And normally, cells also produce antioxidants that neutralize the damaging effects of free radicals, such that a balance is

DOI: http://dx.doi.org/10.5772/intechopen.1004377

created, in this case in the brain, between free radicals and antioxidants. This balance, however, is disrupted by the advent of a traumatic brain injury and can quickly lead to chronic inflammation in the brain. The brain is particularly vulnerable to oxidative stress because brain cells require substantial amounts of oxygen to function properly. Oxidative stress not only disrupts this process but also causes a breakdown of the normal balance between free radicals and antioxidants. In turn, this imbalance can alter essential proteins in the brain, leading to the accumulation of amyloid plaques that eventually lead to neurodegenerative disorders such as Alzheimer's disease, Parkinson's disease, ALS, MS, or chronic traumatic encephalitis (CTE). Here is an example of the progression of neurodegeneration at work, slowly but surely over time. See references [1] and [2] for further information on the process of oxidative stress.

Another example of this neurodegenerative process within Architecture Two: is **glutamate excitotoxicity.** Glutamate excitotoxicity refers to the toxic actions of excitatory neurotransmitters, primarily glutamate. Exacerbated and prolonged activation of glutamate receptors in the brain begins a cascading process of neurotoxicity, leading to the loss of neuronal functioning and cell death, killing part of the neuron through the overactivation of glutamate. Here again, we see the disruption of normal brain/mind functioning, leading to a breakdown of what is normal functioning, and in the case of my patient, leading to his severe symptoms (listed above). See reference [3] for further information on glutamate excitotoxicity.

A third example of the processes of neurodegeneration within Architecture Two is **hyper-perfusion.** This might appear to be a stretch, but let us consider the following. Hyper-perfusion refers to the dysregulated state of blood flow in the brain following the restoration of arterial blood flow to the brain. This is usually considered in the context of treatments for carotid artery stenosis and can be a serious problem because it can lead to severe swelling in the brain, intracranial bleeding, and even death. Hyper-perfusion becomes an issue when the normal mechanisms the brain utilizes for autoregulation (to maintain a constant state of pressure in the brain even when there are changes in blood flow to and within the brain) fail. What I am suggesting here (and this does fall into Architecture Three as well) is that when the brain is traumatized, there are many disruptions to brain/mind functioning. But if this process continues, this cascading neurodegeneration, the brain/mind goes from disruption to breakdown. And hyper-perfusion is an example of how this can happen when autoregulation fails. The brain/mind must maintain a constant, finely tuned balance, that is easy to disrupt and easy to overlook. And this is why I believe we need to recognize, worldwide, how often the brain/mind is involved in illness, disease, and injury and how serious the consequences are when medicine, psychology, and the legal system do not recognize this. Again, the four architectures help us understand the details of this neurodegenerative disease in the brain/mind resulting from trauma to this marvelous organ. See references [4] and [5] for further information on the process of hyper-perfusion in the brain.

4. Back to behavior

Now, turning from biology back to behavior. What can be done to treat Mr. A's symptomatology? No easy task!

Toward this understanding, my patient and I had the following interaction:

Dr. R. "What do you think are the impairments you face as a result of the TBI? At a conference I recently attended it was brought to our attention that understanding the patient's impairments is actually more important than understanding their diagnosis.

We know that you are struggling with a TBI (post-concussion syndrome), but what exactly are the impairments that follow this diagnosis?"

P. "I'm thinking about my college classroom. I easily lose focus and I have difficulty retaining the information I am learning. My process is: lose focus, start to fall behind in the classroom, feel stressed out, and then start to panic."

Dr. R. "Are you ever able to regain your focus in the classroom?"

P. "Not really. I just remain drifting off somewhere. I think I'm dissociating at that point."

Dr. R. "When the brain gets overwhelmed, I believe this is exactly what it does. It dissociates to conserve energy. Or it shuts off through an Absence Seizure, when the person goes totally blank and has no memory of what just happened."

P. "I think I probably am dissociating every class then, right at the point where I start to get overwhelmed."

Dr. R. "What do you think would help you be able to focus better and not dissociate so often?"

R. "You had asked me if I thought our work together was like you providing me with an auxiliary ego. I think it is more accurate for me to say that in our work together you are more like an auxiliary organizer. You help me understand why I am having these problems and what I need to do to fix them."

It is fascinating to me that despite a significant cognitive handicap, Mr. A. was able to use his intellect to find a way around his processing problems, and eventually arrive at a solution to his math and statistics class. It is also fascinating to me that traumatic brain injuries do not diminish the individual's intelligence or consciousness. What is affected is the execution of their intelligence. Further, I agree with Mr. A's point that in our sessions, the doctor functioning as an auxiliary-organizer, is the most accurate description of our work together (as opposed to an auxiliary ego, which is similar but not quite the same). This is why I believe "listening to the brain" and simply being with TBI patients is so crucial to understanding their impairments and doing the repair work. And this is why I find processing the injury, through neuro-psychoanalytic work, so important to the patient's recovery.

In working with TBI patients I use the concept of the "Basket of 4 Symptoms" as a means of organizing the patient's everyday life and organizing our work together during sessions. My patients and I have found the four baskets a very helpful way of organizing their daily lives and their treatment sessions. How well are they doing in each of these areas is a primary concern during each of our sessions.

The four baskets are:

- Physical Symptoms.
- Cognitive Decline.
- Social and Emotional Issues
- Sleep Disturbances.

5. Conclusions

In closing, I want to share a few thoughts about neuro-psychoanalytic theory and practice as being the most effective approach to working with brain-injured patients

DOI: http://dx.doi.org/10.5772/intechopen.1004377

and how this works with the architecture model. Neuro-psychoanalysis is an approach to understanding and treating human behavior that integrates neuroscience and psychoanalysis, mind and brain, brain and mind. I believe the best way to understand brain/mind integration is the conception that the human mind is the subjective experience of the brain.

I noted that neuroscience works through brain imaging, post-mortem dissection, neurological examinations, and testing to understand how the brain functions. And psychoanalysis works through understanding the patient's unconscious agenda, their resistances, and the patient's psychic structure (how they construct both their internal and external worlds). Woven together, neuro-psychoanalysis appreciates that our reality is dependent on the neuro-biological functioning of the brain and our psychological interpretation of this experience.

As is evident in this chapter, I learned a lot about Mr. A's neurological and psychological impairments by listening carefully to his experiences in coping with his post-concussion syndrome. And I was able to do this through having created a physical and psychological space within which he could express his day-to-day experiences. This is the neuro-psychoanalytic approach that allows me to listen effectively to his brain/mind. What he struggled with the most were the issues of cognitive decline (in the four baskets of symptoms), most clearly manifested in Architecture Two (disruptions in electrical and chemical communications in the brain). These disruptions in electrical and chemical communications in the brain led to his struggles with cognitive decline: difficulties with focus, concentration, and attention, decision making, problem solving, memory and easily being overstimulated by his environment at work, and with family and friends. Because the internal "hardware" in his brain was simply not connecting normally.

Finally, listening to my patients over the past 7 years, I developed the following treatment protocol, designed uniquely for each patient, and based on the conception that every TBI is also a person bringing with them their own developmental history, values, ideas, beliefs, conflicts, and motivations that affect the healing process.

1. A pharmacology (I prefer nutrients and supplements to drugs).

2. Stimulating the Brain (I find music with noise-canceling headphones the best way to stimulate healing in the brain).

3. Total Immersion (I have found that demands on the brain for any kind of effort interfere with healing and need to be reduced in favor of reduced demands, physical or mental, on the brain).

4. The Creation of Flow Activities that reduce demands on the brain and allow for healing to occur.

5. Neuro-psychoanalytic sessions that process the injury, and the effects of the injury on the individual's personhood.

Author details

Leighton J. Reynolds
Treatment and Tools for Trauma, Los Angeles, California, United States

*Address all correspondence to: leightonj@sbcglobal.net

References

[1] "How Does Oxidative Stress Affects the Body" by Jamie Eske and medically reviewed by Stacey Sampon. 2019. Available from: https://www.medicalnewstoday.com/articles/324863

[2] "Everything You Should Know About Oxidative Stress" by Megan Dix RN BSN, and medically reviewed by Timothy J. Legg. 2018. Available from: https://www.healthline.com/health/oxidativestress

[3] Kirdajova DB et al. Ischemia-triggered glutamate Excitotoxicity from the perspective of glial cells. Frontiers in Cellular Neuroscience. 2020;**14**:51

[4] "What is Cerebral Hyper-perfusion Syndrome" by Daniel Yetman and medically reviewed by Alana Biggers. 2022. Available from: https://www.healthline.com/hyperfusion

[5] Lin Y-H, Liu H-M. Update on cerebral hyper-perfusion syndrome. Journal of Neuro Interventional Surgery. 2020;**12**(8):788-793. Available from: https://jnis.bmj.com/content/12/8/788

Chapter 2

Diagnosis and Management Process in Traumatic Brain Injury

Pauline N. Kariuki and Motari Omariba

Abstract

Every year, over 10 million people worldwide suffer from traumatic brain injury. A shock, blow, or bump to the head, as well as a penetrating head injury, can all result in traumatic brain damage (TBI), which is a disturbance of normal brain function. It also comes with potential side effects, like oxygen deprivation-induced damage, increased intracranial pressure, and cerebral edema. Traumatic brain damage comes in two primary forms: closed and open. Both primary and secondary effects might result from an injury that is localized (focal injury) or diffuse (widespread). In order to prevent the secondary injuries brought on by conditions like hypoxia and hypotension, management of severe TBI entails receiving acute care with close attention to the airway, oxygenation, and appropriate hemodynamic support. Treating people with traumatic brain injuries remains difficult. Research has made a substantial contribution to our understanding of how injuries occur and how general hospital care is provided. Further research is required to help build evidence-based therapy techniques that can be used to improve functional results and lessen patient management variability.

Keywords: trauma, brain, injury, diagnosis, management

1. Introduction

Each year, traumatic brain injury (TBI) affects over 10 million individuals worldwide. This is according to the World Health Organization's global road safety status report as cited by Hyder et al. [1], which vividly voices the severity of the issue, both currently and in the future, and demonstrates the critical need for well-thought-out assessment plans for prevention, management, and rehabilitation programs. Centers for Disease Control and Prevention (CDC) [2] asserts that TBI is an abnormality in the way the brain normally functions and can be brought on by a blow, jolt, or shock to the head as well as penetrating head injuries. On the other hand, TBI can also result from side effects such cerebral edema and elevated blood pressure that happen after oxygen-related injuries. There are two main types of TBI. These are: closed and open TBI.

IntechOpen

Raskin and Mateer [3] assert that, even in situations when there is not a direct hit to the head, like whiplash, brain damage can still happen. Long-range connecting fibers in the brain may be stretched or even severed by twisting or rotational pressures when the head is abruptly accelerated and decelerated, as in a car collision. When these fibers are damaged, nerve cell communication is hampered, which lowers the effectiveness of large-scale brain networks.

Neurons are the nerve cells that are charged with the responsibility of sending messages all over the body for normal body functions to occur. However, they are weak and are easily destroyed by stretching, cutting, or pressure. An injury to them therefore interferes with signals transmitted to and from the brain causing disruption in communication even in circumstances where there is no direct hit to the head.

In the US, almost 2.8 million individuals are treated in the hospitals annually for TBIs [4]. Based on crude clinical symptoms, including a patient's gross levels of consciousness (e.g., Glasgow Coma Scale (GCS) scores of 13–15), the majority of TBIs are classified as moderate (mTBI). Despite the widely acknowledged possibility of persistent incapacity resulting from moderate to severe TBIs, large-scale brain networks remain effective [5], despite the disagreements regarding the anticipated path of clinical recovery for individuals with mTBI [6]. Even though it has been documented that acute symptoms are typically caused by mTBI [7], and cognitive impairment with challenges in daily functioning [8], however, results differ about whether individuals continue to show signs of mild traumatic brain damage months or years after the incident [9]. Moreover, CDC [2] highlights that TBI continues to be the top cause of mortality in the US for all people aged 1–44, ranks third for those aged 45–64, ranks fifth for newborns under a year old, and ranks seventh for people aged 65 and over. The public health importance of TBI therefore cannot be underestimated.

Large-scale brain networks are graphical representation of brain structure consisting of nodes and edges between pairs of nodes. Some of the brain networks include sensory motor, limbic system, visual system, central executive network (CEN), default mode network (DMN), and salient network.

Severe TBI (sTBI) has traditionally been defined as that presenting with head trauma and brain injury with a post-resuscitation GCS score between 3 and 8, despite existence of other alternative classification schemes. Patients requiring intensive care, often for many days to a few weeks, include those with sTBI and some with so-called mild TBI, defined as a GCS score of 9–12. The initial blow (primary injury) that can cause a variety of structural diseases as well as initiation of chemical, electrical, and inflammatory cascade of physiological events that make up the secondary brain injury are all part of the pathophysiology of traumatic brain injury (TBI). Moreover, the degree of secondary injury sustained and, eventually, the functional result of patients are significantly influenced by secondary insults, including hypotension, hypoxia, seizures, and other physiological events. Patients with sTBI and polytrauma pose a serious risk due to the possibility of persistent secondary insults from vascular and musculoskeletal trauma as well as other organ injuries [10].

The areas of the brain that are prone to secondary hypoxic and hypotensive damage include the hippocampus, thalamus, cerebral cortex, and cerebellum. Some of the clinical signs that manifest include impaired awareness levels, coma, seizures, and stroke. The brain is normally sensitive to hypoxia because of its high energy level requirements compared to the low energy reserves that renders it vulnerable to hypoxic conditions. Hypoxia occurs when there is serious blood loss that leads to low blood pressure or as a result of brain edema that restricts oxygen supply to brain.

2. Categories of TBI

TBI can be classified into three groups based on the distinct physical processes of injury as follows: closed head injury (i), penetrating injury (ii), and explosive blast injury (iii). Some of the clinical signs of traumatic brain injury include prolonged coma, headache, nausea, aphasia, seizures, amnesia, and aberrant behaviors including aggression and anxiety. These symptoms typically manifest seconds to minutes after the injury, although some of them might last for months or even years [11, 12].

Black et al. [13] claim that blunt impact injuries, primarily from road traffic accidents (RTA), falls, and sporting activities are the predominant cause of closed head traumatic brain injuries (TBI). This type of TBI has the highest incidence rate among common people. The brain's regular functioning is disrupted immediately underneath the hit site due to a powerful, blunt contact force that causes compression, directly damaging the brain's vascular and neuronal cells. The authors further note that penetrating traumatic brain injury (TBI) happens when a foreign body enters the skull, passes through the dura, and enters the brain parenchyma. Similar to closed head trauma, localized injuries, intracranial hemorrhage, cerebral edema, and ischemia are the main outcomes of brain tissue laceration.

Experience has shown that young children and the elderly aged over 65 years are more likely to suffer from TBI than other age groups. Risk factors that expose young children to TBI include impaired judgment and poor motor coordination that easily exposes them to unintentional accidents, for example, in instances where they practice to cycle or to skid. The elderly are likely to be exposed due to accidental falls such as in the shower rooms. The falls maybe fatal or may lead to longer periods of hospitalization.

Warden [14] assertions point that the twentieth century saw severe brain damage from combat caused explosive explosions and their consideration in TBI was added as a new category. Ling and Ecklund [15] confirm that, in contrast to closed head injuries and penetrating TBI, the brain is damaged by explosive pressure shock waves that transfer a massive amount of energy from the skull into the enclosed brain parenchyma. They also note that, depending on the outcome of the injury at various stages of the blast-induced injury, the effects of blast injury can be further classified into four patterns: (i) primary (shock wave causing internal damage), (ii) secondary (penetrating), (iii) tertiary (physical injury by blast wave), and, finally, (iv) quaternary (other than the first three classes).

Primary blast-induced injuries result from high pressures arising from flying objects that travel through the body at high velocity from explosives. The strong and fast-moving force can shatter an individual's body and cause massive damage to internal organs such as the kidney, liver, the ears, abdomen, and so on. The secondary blast injuries result from sharp objects and other flying debris carried by strong winds that accompany the primary blast hitting the body causing closed or penetrating injuries. The tertiary blast waves are normally caused by strong pressure gradients accompanied by strong winds that accelerate an individual to hit a solid object such as a stationary vehicle, wall, or other hard surface, just like in typical road traffic accidents (RTAs) resulting in fractured bones, severed limbs, and open or closed injuries on the brain. Quaternary blast injuries occur as a result of other explosive products such as massive heat and toxic substances, for instance, gas or fuels that can cause burns of varied degrees on the body, loss of eyesight, or inhalation of noxious fumes, which can lead to breathing problems.

3. Pathophysiology of TBI

3.1 Primary brain injuries

Risdall and Menon [16] observe that there are two types of damage to the neuronal tissues linked to TBI: (i) primary injury, which is directly brought on by mechanical forces during the initial insult, and (ii) secondary injury, which is defined as additional tissue and cellular damages that occur after the primary insult.

Skandsen et al. [17] note that focal and diffuse brain injuries are the two main forms of primary injuries that can result from the initial impact of various mechanical assaults to the brain. Research findings indicate that patients with moderate to severe traumatic brain injury frequently have both types of damage concurrently. However, Schmidt et al. [18] write that about 70% of cases of traumatic brain injury (TBI) are caused by diffuse axonal damage (DAI). Closed head TBI and penetrating TBI show focal brain damage with signs of a fractured skull and localized contusion in the center of the injury site as a result of lacerations, compressions, and concussion forces.

Hemiparesis, behavioral abnormalities, and cognitive disabilities might result from an injury, depending on its severity. Unlike focal injury, diffuse brain injury is mostly caused by noncontact forces of fast acceleration and deceleration, which injure the cerebral brain tissues by shearing and stretching them. Strong tensile strains harm blood vessels, oligodendrocytes, and neuronal axons, resulting in ischemic brain injury and brain edema [19].

Hemiparesis is one the most common effect of TBI. Its presentation depends on the severity of the TBI. The more severe the TBI, the more severe the loss of motor control, in which case it is referred to as hemiplegia (paralysis on either the right or left side of the body) as opposed to hemiparesis (weakness on either the right or left side of the body). TBI can cause behavioral abnormalities due to changes on how the brain functions. There may be some dysregulation in an individual's personality as well as an increased risk of depression. Experience has shown that patients with moderate to severe TBI normally suffer from a range of long-term neurocognitive consequences such as memory loss, loss of executive functions, and attention deficits.

3.2 Secondary brain injuries

The physiological, cellular, and biochemical processes that take place during a primary injury can result in secondary damages that are delayed and extended and can endure for hours or years. Mechanistically, excitotoxicity, mitochondrial dysfunction, oxidative stress, lipid peroxidation, neuroinflammation, axon degeneration, and apoptotic cell death are some of the causes that lead to secondary injuries [20].

Figure 1 (on the left) portrays diagrammatic representation of physiology of TBI. It shows how an increase in cell adhesion molecules facilitates activated leukocyte transmigration into the damaged brain parenchyma as a result of blood-brain barrier (BBB) due to traumatic brain injury.

Reactive oxygen species (ROS) and inflammatory chemicals including chemokines and cytokines are produced by activated leukocytes, microglia, and astrocytes and can impair neuronal activity by causing demyelination, axonal cytoskeleton disruption, axonal swelling, and an accumulation of transport proteins at the terminals.

Neurodegeneration results in progressive axonal injury. Further, glial scar development brought on by astrogliosis at the lesion site produces an environment that is nonpermissive and inhibits axonal regeneration. However, glutamate-induced

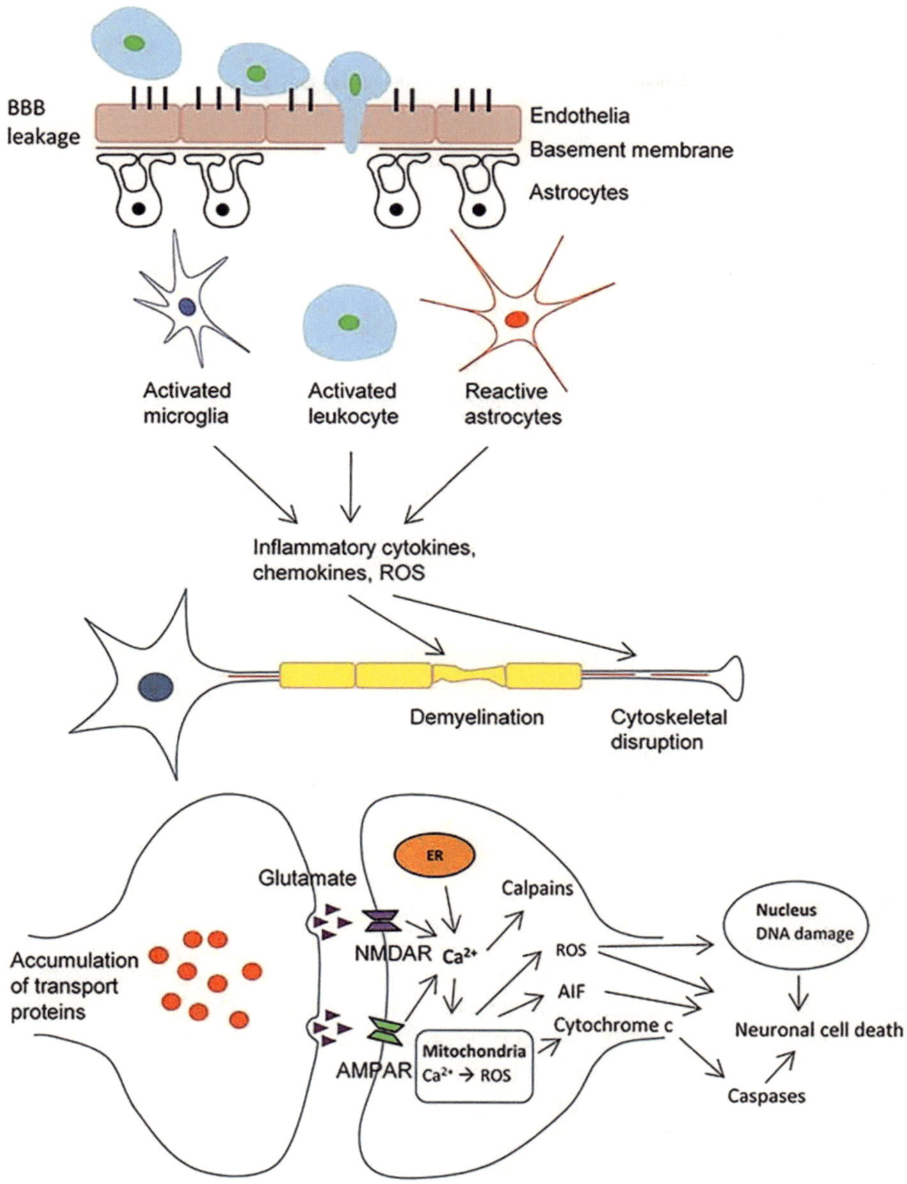

Figure 1.
Schematic representation of pathophysiology of TBI.

aggravated release from presynaptic nerve terminals, excessive accumulation of glutamate and aspartate neurotransmitters in the synaptic space as a result of spillage from severed neurons, and impaired reuptake mechanisms in traumatic and ischemic brain activate N-methyl-d-aspartate (NMDA) and α-amino-3-hydroxy-5-methyl-4-isoxazolepropionic acid (AMDA) receptors on postsynaptic membranes, allowing calcium ions to enter. These processes cause the release of Ca^{2+} ions from the endoplasmic reticulum (ER), an intracellular storage, which in turn causes the generation of reactive oxygen species (ROS) and the activation of capillaries. Molecules including cytochrome c and apoptosis-inducing factor (AIF) are released into the cytosol due to mitochondrial malfunction. Neuronal cell death that is both caspase-dependent and -independent is the result of these cellular and molecular processes, which also involve the interaction of Fas and Fas ligand [20].

4. Diagnosis of TBI

Teasdale and Jennett [10] recommend that assessment and treatment of TBI should be done concurrently, starting with the ABC, that is, airway, breathing/respiration, and then circulation. Next, D should follow. The D component includes assessment and management of neurological status. As part of the motor examination, patients' responsiveness to eye opening, motor activity, and speech is evaluated, and a GCS score is given both before and after resuscitation. It is important to take note of any lateralizing signals, which are significant indicators of presence of a concomitant spinal cord injury or cerebral lesions as well as a neurologic deficit along the spinal cord which can be determined through neurologic examination. After GCS had been documented, lateralizing signs that should be examined that include checking for symmetry in pupil of the eyes and their response to light, movement in the all the upper and lower extremities, planter reflexes, and deep tendon reflexes. If the pupils are unequal, it signals lateralizing motor weakness. Muscle power in the extremities will indicate if there is any indication of paralysis. A disruption of the corticospinal and other descending pathways that affect the reflex arc resulting from a suprasegmental lesion is indicated by abnormal deep tendon reflexes. A structural or metabolic anomaly in the corticospinal system above the segmental reflex will be indicated by an aberrant planter reflex.

4.1 Glasgow coma scale (GCS)

The GCS has been in use for many years. It has a good predictive value for mortality and morbidity in large populations in addition to its high inter-rater reliability. TBI treatment outcome relies on the post-resuscitation score. Special emphasis needs to be on motor assessment during patient examination due to its sensitivity in patients with TBI. However, depending on the type of structural injury, relative degree of secondary injury burden, the emergence of neurologic or systemic complications, and other known and unknown genetic and epigenetic factors, patient presenting with a particular GCS scores may ultimately have a wide range of outcomes. The goal of treatment therefore is to maximize the healing environment by reducing harmful and disabling events. It is imperative to promptly conduct a thorough survey of traumatic findings related to traumatic brain injury (**Table 1** and **Figure 2**) [21].

The GCS helps medical providers determine how conscious (or how deeply in a coma) one is based on eye, speech, and movement responses. Davanzo et al. [22] recommend that traumatic findings associated with TBI should include the pupils, cranium, eyes, ears and nose, face, and neck.

4.1.1 Pupils

Other neurological signs include pupil size, symmetry, and reactivity. Anomalies in these areas are useful in identifying whether or not a brain herniation necessitating immediate medical attention is present. However, they are also linked to other types of trauma, such as direct damage to the globe, direct injury to the oculomotor nerve,

GCS aggregate score ranges between 3 and 15. The results of each test (E for eye, V for verbal, and M for motor) are reported as the GCS.

Test	Not testable (NT): examples	1	2	3	4	5	6
Eye response	Severity of injury to the eyes, enucleation	Eyes closed	Eyes open in reaction to discomfort	Eyes open in reaction to voice	Spontaneously opens eyes	Not applicable	Not applicable
Verbal response	Indwelling tube, not able to talk, language barrier	Silent	Incomprehensible sounds	Inappropriate words	Confused and disoriented, but able to answer question	Oriented to time, person, and place, converses normally	Not applicable
Motor response	Paralysis/hemiparesis (acquired causes such as post-stroke, post-neurological injury; congenital/innate such as cerebral palsy)	Makes no movements	Abnormal extension (decerebrate posture)	Abnormal flexion (decorticate posture)	Flexion/withdrawal from painful stimuli	Moves to localize pain	Obeys commands

Table 1.
Glasgow Coma Scale developed by Teasdale and Jennett [21].

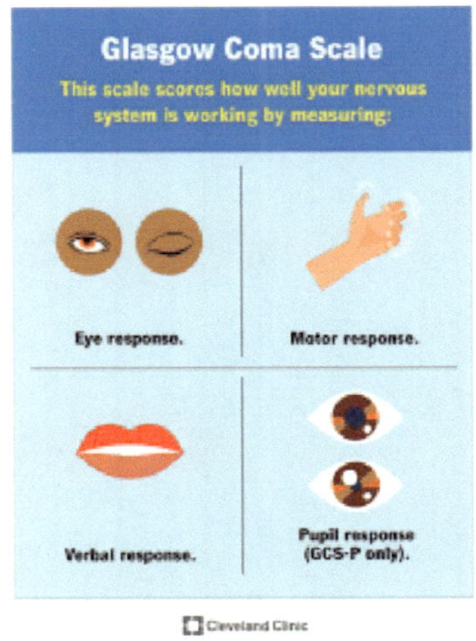

Figure 2.
GCS assessment (Source: Cleveland Clinic).

or blunt vascular injury (Horner syndrome) (as opposed to the compression brought on by a herniated brain) [22]. Brain herniation among patients with traumatic brain injury can be detected through pupil examination. It maybe indicated when the pupil(s) is dilated and may not narrow in response to light. However, brain herniation can also be detected through CT scan and MRI. The most common brain herniation is subfalcine hernia also called midline shift or cingulate hernia.

4.1.2 Cranium

Signs of head and neck trauma must be examined for after the quick neurologic examination and GCS score are determined. In order to accurately assess the type and degree of scalp abrasions, contusions, and lacerations as well as the existence of open depressed skull fractures within lacerations, it may necessary to shave the head to necessitate physical examination. Basilar skull fractures are frequently linked to the occurrence of bilateral periorbital ecchymoses, also known as raccoon eyes, or mastoid ecchymoses, also known as Battle's sign. It is important to feel the calvarium for abnormalities that could indicate closed skull fractures [22]. Raccoon eyes, another name for Battle's sign, are characterized by a broad bruise that covers the entire back of the ears and sometimes even reaches the top of the neck. Battle's sign patients can develop raccoon eyes, which is a term for ocular bruises associated with a skull fracture.

4.1.3 Eyes

As soon as patients are able to obey commands, extraocular motions should be evaluated since cranial nerve palsies might result from initial damage to the nuclei, compression within the cranium, or impingement in the orbit. A fixed gaze among BTI patients could indicate nonconvulsive seizure activity or status epilepticus. Important danger signs (indicators) like subconjunctival hemorrhage or hyphemia, which are usually considered as ophthalmologic emergencies, should be reported immediately after they are spotted. These may be signs of hypoxemia and direct trauma to the globe and conjunctival petechiae [22]. A buildup of blood in the anterior chamber of the eyes is called hyphemia. This is the typical point of entry and exit for fluid that nourishes the tissues around the eye. Blunt trauma is the most common cause of hyphemia.

4.1.4 Ears and nose

When hemotympanum or external auditory canal hemorrhage is observed during an otoscopic examination, the source and any related injuries (such as a fractured skull, a ruptured tympanic membrane, or damage to the ossicles and other ear structures) should be carefully checked for and managed. The presence of cerebrospinal fluid (CSF), otorrhea, or rhinorrhea indicates a fracture to the base of the skull and a dural laceration. It also increases the chances of BTI patients developing meningitis later on. Nonetheless, the majority of CSF leaks linked to skull base fractures resolve on their own and do not need to be treated. The patient therefore needs frequent observations to monitor their progress [22]. If the depression is more than 5 mm below the inner table of the adjacent bone, elevating the depressed skull fracture is the recommended surgical treatment for dural laceration and base of the skull fracture. Reducing contamination is the indication for elevation.

4.1.5 Face

Soft tissue injuries and concurrent face fractures are common among BTI patients. Their nature of presentation can therefore influence the choice of surgery. Therefore, a very comprehensive evaluation of these injuries is required, along with imaging if necessary and careful repair and management of any bleeding that may be present. Craniofacial bone structural integrity is necessary for maintaining cranial integrity after numerous fractures. However, the presence of brain edema frequently causes fracture repair to be delayed; therefore, surgical techniques need to be coordinated among doctors [22]. As soon as brain edema subsides, the multidisciplinary surgical team can then coordinate and commence any surgical and or conservative treatment that maybe needed to improve the patients' recovery process.

4.1.6 Neck

Watridge et al. [23] observe that in the following clinical circumstances, concomitant blunt vascular injury (BVI) may occur and should therefore be considered.

- A neurological deficiency in the brain that is not evidenced through computed tomography (CT).
- Monoparesis in conscious individuals who are not diagnosed with brachial plexus injury
- Lucid interval followed by a decline in neurologic function
- Unexplained dysphasia
- One sided headache after the injury

- Arterial nose-bleeding
- Horner syndrome resulting from damage of some pathways in the sympathetic nervous system causing ptosis, miosis, anhidrotic, and so forth
- Evidence of bleeding in the neck that may result from blunt neck trauma among the BTI patients neck hematoma, ecchymosis resulting from blood leaking from broken blood vessels into the tissues of the skin or mucus membranes or crepitus resulting from gas in soft tissues.

Anecdotal evidence suggests that other clinical signs noted in such patients include spasticity, which may set in 1 week after injury that maybe evidenced through hypertonicity and spasms of the affected muscles and exaggerated deep tendon reflexes.

Biffl et al. [24] caution that some of obvious risk factors for blunt cerebrovascular injury are:

Cervical injury resulting from its overextension with rotation:

- GCS rated at 8 or below
- Neck, hanging, or strangulation or mechanical injuries caused by seatbelts
- Fractures of the base of the skull, particularly into the carotid canal or foramen lacerum
- Fractures of the face specifically Le Fort II and III
- Fracture of the cervical spine
- Other injuries of vascular nature, for instance, thoracic aorta.

Miller et al. [25] recommend that the multidisciplinary team involved in the management of TBI patients should be keen and examine for any possible blunt vascular injury (BVI) because traumatic cervical artery dissection, thromboembolism, and occlusion are preventable secondary insults to the brain that can cause large areas of ischemia, which can be fatal in addition to increasing the burden of neurologic deficits.

5. Cognitive challenges after TBI

Cognitive function has been defined as "the mental action or process of acquiring knowledge and understanding through thought, experience, and senses" [26]. It includes processes such as knowledge, attention, memory and working memory, judgment and assessment, reasoning and "computation," problem-solving and decision-making, comprehension, and language production. Studies indicate that cognitive functions create new knowledge by applying preexisting knowledge. Following a traumatic brain injury, cognitive dysfunction, which includes issues with planning, problem-solving, attention, and timing, and cognitive-behavioral and psycho-behavioral disorders are common symptoms. After a traumatic brain injury, persistent memory loss and executive function impairment are also prevalent [27].

Experience shows that BTI patients lose both long- and short-term memories. It is commonly observed that such patients present with short term memory seen through trouble grasping and remembering new information, what happens on day-to-day basis as well as recalling recent events that have occurred.

Lennon et al. [28] argue that, although controversial debates still exist on the exact cognitive domains most affected by TBI, there is consensus that TBI produces cognitive impairment. However, investigations of mild-to-severe TBI reveal a higher mixture of positive and negative results, despite the fact that moderate-to-severe TBI is considered to be harmful to the patients. Lennon et al. [28] conducted a study that looked at the number of mTBIs and the severity of TBIs in later life and their longer-term cognitive effects. The study employed a subgroup ($n = 15{,}764$) of the PROTECT, a cohort that evaluated risk factors for cognitive impairment in people between the ages of 50 and 90. For 4 years, participants underwent cognitive tests annually. Principal component analysis (PCA) was used to categorize the results of cognitive tests into working memory, episodic memory, attention, processing speed, and executive function. Participants used the Brain Injury Screening Questionnaire (BISQ) to retrospectively recollect the number and severity of TBIs they had experienced over their lifetime. The impact of head injury severity (non-TBI head hit, mTBI, and moderate-severe TBI) and the number of mTBI at baseline and throughout time were investigated using linear mixed models (LMMs). mTBI was divided into five groups: 0 mTBI, 1 mTBI, 2 mTBIs, 3 mTBIs, and 4+ mTBIs. It was regarded as a continuous and categorical variable. Of the individuals, 3711 (23.5%) had at most experienced a non-TBI head impact, 510 (3.2%) had at least one moderate-severe TBI, and 5725 (36.3%) had no head injuries at all. The average standard deviation (SD) of the individuals' most recent reported head injury was 29.6 (20.0) years ago before the study began. In terms of results, longitudinal cognitive trajectories did not worsen across the course of the trial, but there were notable cognitive abnormalities linked to TBI at baseline.

Individuals with at least one moderate-severe traumatic brain injury (TBI) at baseline showed significantly lower executive scores ($B = 0.151$, $p = 0.004$), processing speed ($B = 0.075$, $p = 0.033$), and attention ($B = -0.163$, $p < 0.001$). At baseline, the group with at least one mTBI showed significantly lower attention scores than the group without a head injury ($B = -0.052$, $p = 0.001$). The individuals in the 3 mTBI group showed lower baseline executive function ($B = -0.149$, $p = 0.025$) and attention scores ($B = -0.085$, $p = 0.015$) in comparison to those without mTBI. When compared to individuals who reported no mTBI, those who had experienced four or more mTBIs at baseline showed worse attention ($B = -0.135$, $p < 0.001$), processing speed ($B = -0.072$, $p = 0.009$), and working memory ($B = -0.052$, $p = 0.036$). Cognitive deficits related to traumatic brain injury are dose-, fixed-, and severity-dependent. When compared to working memory and processing speed, the effects of attention and executive function are almost twice as strong, making them the most sensitive cognitive domains. According to their recommendations, domain-specific effects should be properly targeted in post-TBI cognitive rehabilitation. Furthermore, having three or more lifetime mTBIs was linked to significant long-term cognitive abnormalities. This is important to keep in mind when counseling people who have had a TBI against continuing high-risk activities.

Teasdale and Jennett [10] note that the incidence estimates for sTBI, which are based on a GCS of 3–6, are significantly lower, at 4–6/100,000/year. Nonetheless, because of the significant functional impact of the injuries and the personal pain that patients and their families endure, sTBI is a serious health issue. The spectrum of deficits and impairments associated with severe traumatic brain injuries varies in complexity, potentially impacting an individual's physical and emotional well-being.

Anecdotal evidence suggests that some of the deficits and impairments include impaired consciousness with post-traumatic amnesia. Physical deficits include loss of balance and coordination, difficulties in ambulation, loss of fine motor skills and loss of strength, and lack of exercise tolerance, while cognitive deficits include difficult in communication and information processing with altered perceptual skills. Patients with TBI are urged to use memory aids such notepads, daily task lists, calendars, schedules, and reminder apps as part of their cognitive rehabilitation. In addition, they must regularly practice newly learned material, manage their anxieties, and get adequate sleep.

Dahm and Ponsford [29] note that it has been demonstrated that, throughout time, neurobehavioral and cognitive deficits have a greater total disability following TBI than physical impairments.

6. Treatment goals

Goal-directed TBI treatment should include maintaining certain clinical considerations. While some of the objectives, like cerebral perfusion pressure (CPP), intracranial pressure (ICP), and continuous brain tissue oxygenation ($PbtO_2$) monitoring are particularly pertinent to patients receiving care in an intensive care unit (ICU), maintaining normocapnia and adequate oxygenation is crucial to all other BTI patients. Pulmonary-specific characteristics may be necessary for patients with severe respiratory problems (such as acute respiratory distress syndrome). To prevent hypotension, it is important to regularly monitor both mean arterial pressure and systolic blood pressure (SBP). Regular temperature monitoring is important in TBI patients to maintain normothermia at 38°C [30].

Electrolytes should be kept within a typical range. It is critical to pay close attention to the salt level to avoid hyponatremia in TBI patients since it can exacerbate cerebral edema. It has been observed that if electrolytes are not kept within normal levels, they can trigger serious health problems such as kidney problems, hypertension, and cardiac arrythmias. Patients with traumatic brain injury may also experience the syndrome of inappropriate antidiuretic hormone (SIADH) or diabetes insipidus (DI). Patients' serum sodium and osmolality levels should be checked often. Hypoglycaemia and hyperglycaemia can have a negative impact on TBI patients' prognosis. Every TBI patient needs to have their serum glucose levels regularly checked. After nutritional therapy is started, more frequent monitoring is necessary, especially for patients with known or suspected diabetes mellitus [30].

Anemia and abnormal coagulation are common in patients with TBI, thus should be strictly monitored. However, there is considerable practice variability in hemoglobin transfusion thresholds for TBI patients. A recent randomized clinical research examined two thresholds for hemoglobin transfusion following traumatic brain injury (7 and 10 g/dl). The neurological result was the same in both cases. The 10 g/dl barrier however was linked to a higher frequency of adverse outcomes, bolstering the 7 g/dl transfusion threshold suggested as best practices. In order to identify medical, iatrogenic, or early posttraumatic coagulopathy when present, TBI patients should have early screening for coagulopathy, including testing for direct and indirect coagulation cascades using the international normalized ratio (INR). The use of more recent coagulation capacity testing (such as platelet function assays, thromboelastography,

≥ 95% in pulse oximetry	ICP between 20 and 25 mmHg	Sodium in serum, 135–145
PaO_2 < 100 mmHg	$PbtO_2$ < 15 mmHg	INR less than 1.4
$PaCO_2$ between 35 and 45 mmHg	CPP more than 60 mmHg	Platelets less than 75 × 103/ mm^3
SBP greater than or equal to 100 mmHg	Temperature between 36.0 and 38°C	> 7 g/dl of hemoglobin
PH 7.35–7.45	Blood sugar 80–180 mg/dL	

*Key: PaO_2: partial oxygen pressure; $PaCO_2$: partial pressure of carbon dioxide; SBP: blood pressure in systolic form; ICP: internal cerebral pressure; $PbtO_2$: oxygen tension in brain tissue; CPP: cerebral perfusion pressure; INR: international normal ratio; * based on the state of brain auto-regulation.*

Table 2.
Goals of treatment.

or rotational thromboelastometry) may yield more information about the necessity of focused therapy to reverse coagulopathy (**Table 2**) [30].

7. Management of traumatic brain injury

7.1 Prehospital management

There are two main categories for TBI: primary and secondary brain injuries. Primary brain injury is the outcome of kinetic energy transfer causing damage to brain tissue. The phrase "secondary brain injury" refers to the worsening of traumatic brain injury (TBI) over the course of minutes to hours due to a variety of circumstances, including hypoxemia, hypotension, hypo- or hypercarbia, hypo- or hyperglycaemia, hypo- or hyperthermia, and seizures. The main goal of therapeutic measures after traumatic brain injury (TBI) is to prevent further brain injury, which is best handled by specialists such as the anesthesiologist, preferably neuro-anesthesiologist [31]. In order to protect the patient's airway and ensure proper breathing and circulation, care for a patient with a traumatic brain injury should start as soon as possible after the damage (**Table 3**) [32].

As soon as feasible, patients with moderate or severe TBI should be sent to a tertiary referral care facility equipped with neurosurgical facilities. Transport techniques, distance from tertiary referral care facility, duration of travel to the tertiary referral care facility, and whether a doctor or a paramedic leads the responding team have all been demonstrated to affect the outcomes for TBI patients. The principal objectives of therapy are to prevent hypoxia and hypotension, as even a moment of hypotension has been linked to a two-fold increase in mortality and a heightened risk of morbidity [33].

7.2 Neurological assessment

Since Teasdale and Jennett's 1974 [10] initial publication of the most popular technique, the GCS, it has been found useful in documenting patients' state of consciousness during initial assessment and in later evaluations. Nonetheless, some authors have challenged the GCS, claiming that it has low interobserver variability, which results in a limited prognostic value. Scales such as Full Outline of Unresponsiveness score and the Simplified Motor Score have been developed as potential enhancements to the GCS, despite controversies. Despite having a better interobserver reliability, they are nevertheless not widely used [34].

Control of breathing and oxygenation
Treatment, diagnosis, and prevention of hypoxia (O_2 saturation less than 90% and/or cyanosis). Maintain constantly high-flow of oxygen for every possible case of TBI
↓
Maneuvers to realign the airways are carried out
↓
When doing bag-valve-mask (BVM) ventilation, airway adjuncts such as an oropharyngeal airway are used
↓
If a qualified ALS provider is present, endotracheal intubation is carried out
Controlling ventilation
• For intubated patients, the goal for $ETCO_2$ is 40 mmHg, and it should be carefully maintained between 35 and 45 mmHg. Aim to keep ventilation rates at the following levels: Breath rates for babies are 25/min, children are 20/min, and adults and adolescents are 10/min. *Mechanical ventilation*: Ventilators will be utilized to maximize O_2 treatment and ventilation parameters when they are available. In order to keep the $ETCO_2$ within the goal range, the target tidal volume should be 6–7 ml/kg, with rates adjusted accordingly.
• *Mode of breathing in case of a brain herniation*: Even in cases of severe brain injury, recommendations for early TBI therapy (prehospital/emergency department) explicitly advise against any "prophylactic hyperventilation" due to compelling evidence against it.
• Only when there are clear indications of a herniation, use recommended guidelines for hyperventilation. It is advised to only mildly hyperventilate in such circumstances. Between 30 and 35 mmHg is the $ETCO_2$ goal range during "mild therapeutic hyperventilation."
Control of blood pressure
• Low blood pressure (*hypotension*): SBP < 90 mmHg has been utilized in the majority of TBI research to diagnose hypotension in adults and older children. Hypotension is defined by the pediatric guidelines as an SBP that is lower than the fifth percentile for the age. The calculation for this is [70 mmHg + (age × 2)].
• *Treatment for low blood pressure*: SBP ≥ 90 mmHg is advised according to TBI recommendations. Intravenous (IV) fluid resuscitation will be started with an initial bolus of 1 L of normal saline or Ringer's lactate in adults and adolescents, and 20 ml/kg in older children, upon a single SBP measurement of less than 90 mmHg. IV fluid treatment at a rate and volume sufficient to sustain SBP ≥ 90 mmHg will follow.
• *Treatment of high blood pressure (hypertension)*: It is not advised to treat acute hypertension in TBI patients. However, in patients with SBP ≥ 140 mmHg, IV fluids will be limited to a modest "keep open" rate.

Table 3.
Protocols for prehospital management [32].

7.3 Management of the Airway and Ventilation

Hypoxemia's unfavorable results have been linked in a number of researches. Studies indicate that TBI patients who were intubated at the scene of trauma had worse results, even though airway control may be our main priority in these individuals [35]. Experience has shown that intubation outside the hospital is a complex and delicate procedure that can expose BTI patients to fatal outcomes resulting from hypoxia, hypotension, or hypertension. Outcomes in such patients are worse especially those who are far from static healthcare facilities.

Preferable anesthetics are those that provide hemodynamic stability, prevent an increase in intracranial pressure (ICP), and enable quick control of the airway.

The most often prescribed medications are thiopental and propofol, though both might result in hypotension. Although etomidate offers benefits for cardiovascular stability, there are chances that it may decrease adrenal function. Ketamine is often prescribed to trauma victims, though recent studies indicate that its impact on ICP is limited [36].

7.4 Blood pressure and cerebral perfusion pressure (CPP)

Vasopressors are frequently used to increase CPP in the context of TBI, despite the fact that there is little information about these medications. Studies indicate that dopamine use results in increased ICP levels, whereas norepinephrine has a more constant and predictable influence on CPP [37]. To reduce mortality and improve outcomes, it is recommended to maintain SBP at ≥100 mmHg for patients 50–69 years old, or at ≥110 mmHg or higher for patients 15–49 or older than 70. Recommended mmHg level is between 60 and 70 mmHg, which is the recommended target CPP value for survival and favorable outcomes. It is uncertain what the lowest ideal CPP threshold is—60 or 70 mmHg—and it might depend on the patient's autonomic state [31].

7.5 Fluid management

First and foremost, hypovolemia from extracranial hemorrhage should be checked out in a patient with hypotensive TBI. Transcapillary leakage can cause hypovolemia even in the absence of extracranial hemorrhage. The degree of hypovolemia can be roughly determined using established techniques, such as assessments of the arterial pulse pressure fluctuation, blood pressure response after a fluid challenge, or a passive leg raise, even though it may be difficult to give accurate results. Research studies appear to indicate that the amount of fluid infused irrespective of the fluid type affects the outcome after traumatic brain injury [31].

7.6 Sedation and analgesia

A key element in the treatment of traumatic brain injury is lowering stress and the adrenocortical response [38]. Due to this stress reaction, even TBI patients who are unconscious may have elevated ICP and blood pressure. By lowering cerebral metabolism and oxygen consumption in a dose-dependent manner, sedative medications might lessen metabolic stress on recently injured brain tissue. This lowers cerebral blood flow (CBF), which lowers intracranial pressure (ICP). Throughout the period of sedation, care should be taken to maintain an appropriate mean arterial pressure [39].

7.7 ICP monitoring and management

It has been demonstrated that patients with raised ICP have worse outcomes and are more likely to die [40]. It has been observed that raised ICP among such patients may lead to severe headache and pressure that may cause severe damage to the brain, restrict blood flow to the brain, and worsen brain herniation leading to severe disruption of brain function.

According to the most recent version of the Brain Trauma Foundation (BTF) guidelines, the following are the indications of ICP monitoring in TBI: (i) ICP monitoring-based treatment of severe traumatic brain injury patients may lower in-hospital and two-week post-injury mortality; (ii) the guidelines no longer provide guidance on which patients should be selected for follow-up due to a lack of high-quality data; and (iii) when a patient is at a high risk of experiencing a clinical deterioration, intracranial monitoring should be started using clinical judgment. BTF guidelines recommend that treating an ICP with more than 22 mmHg can lower mortality, and ICP monitoring is recommended at level IIB. Standardized techniques employing an increasing treatment intensity in a "staircase approach" are part of the management of elevated ICP as shown in **Figure 3**.

In contrast, a three-tiered strategy is suggested by the American College of Surgeons' (AMCS) TBI Guidelines for the treatment of elevated ICP [41]. The standard operation procedure of ICP monitoring is invasive monitoring with the external ventricular drain (EVD) approach, which involves inserting a catheter through a burr hole into one of the ventricles. This method can be used to measure ICP as well as drain CSF and deliver medication intrathecally, such as an antibiotic for ventriculitis patients. Placing an EVD may also be necessary to drain post-traumatic bleeding. An ICP monitor is useful when ICP monitoring is required when there is no need to drain CSF, for example, in instances where there is need to investigate chronic headache. Consequently, at this point, modest drops in CSF can have a significant effect on ICP control. Similarly, craniectomy and duraplasty, which enlarge the cerebral compartment and remove mass lesions, can efficiently manage intracranial pressure [10].

Depending on the amount of space that hemorrhagic lesions and cerebral edema occupy in the intracranial compartment, managing intracranial pressure (ICP) can be quite challenging. According to the Monroe Kellie theory, cerebral tissue, cerebral blood, and CSF all have fixed volumes inside the intracranial compartment. To keep the ICP normal, compensation must take place when the volume of one compartment rises or a mass lesion is added to the compartment. The first step in this adjustment is the movement of venous blood and CSF into the spinal canal. However, when cerebral compliance declines and elastance rises after a critical volume is reached in the intra-cranial compartment, this leads to greater changes in ICP and less changes in volume.

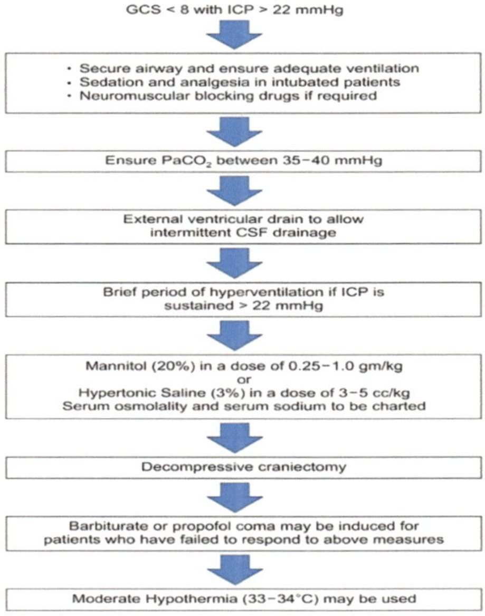

Figure 3.
Stepladder approach to the management of intracranial hypertension (ICP > 22 mmHg) after severe TBI (GCS < 8).

7.8 Osmotherapy

Since the 1960s, mannitol for osmotherapy has been the primary treatment for elevated ICP, and it is still included in TBI management protocols. For the past 20 years, hypertonic saline has gained popularity as an alternative treatment of choice; nevertheless, disagreements among TBI management specialists still exist on the ideal agent and delivery system. Mannitol promotes osmotic diuresis, lowers blood viscosity through distorted erythrocytes, and raises CBF by expanding plasma. By increasing the plasma volume, hypertonic saline facilitates the passage of water across the blood-brain barrier and enhances blood flow. Equiosmolar dosages of hypertonic saline and mannitol were compared by Cottenceau and his research associates for the treatment of elevated ICP. Human subjects treated with hypertonic saline experienced a considerably greater drop in baseline ICP compared to those treated with mannitol [31, 42].

7.9 Multimodal neuro-monitoring

The brain oxygen supply and absorption balance can be estimated using jugular vein oxygen saturation ($SjvO_2$). To reduce contamination from extracranial venous return, a catheter is advanced to the jugular bulb by being placed into the prominent internal jugular vein. A fall in jugular SvO_2 levels below 55% suggests that cerebral oxygen demand may not be sufficient, typically as a result of vasoconstriction linked to hyperventilation or diminished CPP. On the other hand, elevated $SjvO_2$ signifies excessive perfusion occurring due to elevated CBF or reduced oxygen consumption as a result of cell death. After TBI, lower $SjvO_2$ levels (less than 50%) and higher $SjvO_2$ levels (more than 75%) are usually danger signs that are linked to worse outcomes. After a traumatic brain injury, regular $SjvO_2$ monitoring may produce better results [43].

7.10 Anticonvulsant therapy

Convulsive activity after TBI raises intracranial pressure and modifies the flow of oxygen to the wounded brain. Numerous studies have sought to investigate the benefits of seizure prevention in order to prevent subsequent brain injury. Research findings indicate that phenytoin medication was successful in reducing the incidence of post-traumatic seizures during the initial 7 days following injury; however, it did not have a meaningful impact in preventing post-traumatic seizures beyond the first week following injury [44].

7.11 Control of temperature

Temperatures can cause more edema and inflammation; even moderate hyperthermia has been linked in clinical practice to worse results and longer hospitalizations especially in the intensive care unit for patients with traumatic brain injury. On the other hand, cooling has been observed to enhance outcomes after global brain hypoxia and may even be neuroprotective. Because of impaired circulation and hypoxia in the penumbra zone, the damaged brain is very vulnerable to the adrenergic stress brought on by the brain injury itself, which might worsen with active hypothermia [31, 45].

7.12 Control of glycaemia

Following TBI, there is a notable increase in catecholamines, cortisol release, and glucose intolerance that results in significant hyperglycemia. Cerebral edema and neuronal dysfunction may emerge from the brain's acidotic state brought on by anaerobic glucose metabolism. Hyperglycemia after traumatic brain injury has also been linked to impaired cerebrovascular control and poor outcomes. Avoid glucose-containing liquids and keeping an eye on patients' blood sugar levels to keep them between 4 and 8 mmol/L [46].

7.13 Decompressive craniectomy

A decompressive craniectomy is a surgical technique in which a significant portion of the skull is removed. By providing more room for the enlarged brain, a craniectomy lowers ICP and may immediately stop brainstem herniation [31]. Postoperative management includes avoiding exertion for at least 4 weeks after surgery, advising patients to do mild active exercises to maintain joint range of motion, and keeping the surgical site clean. Once regular exercise routine commences and patients complain of headache or fatigue, reducing the amount of exercises and gradually building tolerance is advised.

7.14 Nutrition support

Better results are linked to early nutritional supplementation and enteral feeding has been shown to be advantageous. The BTF advises basal calorie replacement between the 5th and 7th day following injury. Additionally, transgastric jejunal feeding may lower the incidence of pneumonia linked to ventilator use. Patients suffering from sTBI may experience difficulty with stomach emptying due to elevated ICP and opioid use. Metoclopramide is one example of a prokinetic drug that may enhance feeding tolerance [31].

7.15 Antibiotic therapy

Patients with TBIs are more likely to require intrusive monitoring and therapeutic interventions, such as mechanical ventilation, which increases their risk of infection. It is important to locate possible infection sources and start the right treatment [31]. Invasive ICP monitoring is a common source of infection, and it has been observed that the frequency of ICP device infections varies between 1% and 27% [47].

CDC [2] argues that in order to prevent further harm from hypoxia and hypotension, treatment for TBI should involve intensive care, with a focus on the airway, oxygenation, and adequate hemodynamic support. Close monitoring in intensive care for TBI patients is important in order to avoid some of the secondary injuries that may be associated with hypoxia and hypotension. Combined effect of hypoxia and hypotension has been associated with high rates of mortalities among patients with TBI. It is also important to note that adequate ventilation strategy should be in place especially in the 24 hours after traumatic brain injury so that cerebral oxygen delivery is adequately monitored through either jugular oxygen saturation (SjO_2) or brain oxygen tension ($PbrO_2$).

Teasdale and Jennett [10] confirm that as soon as first responders assess a patient with sTBI, treatment must start. In order to improve long-term outcomes after sTBI, emergency personnel and physicians in multiple specialties need to be knowledgeable about the diagnosis and treatment of sTBI. This includes minimizing secondary cerebral injury, promptly coordinating surgical care for structural injuries requiring surgery, and preventing secondary insults to the greatest extent possible.

TBI patients may present with brain damage that is structural in nature that results from the main injury. Effects of the structural damage must therefore be lessened.

When treating a range of structural injuries, surgery is frequently performed either early (for compressive lesions pressing on the brain) or later (for example, when treating CSF leaks or infections, treating developing cerebral edema, and performing craniofacial repairs). Extra-axial mass lesions are located outside the brain tissue but inside the cranium, whereas intra-axial mass lesions are located within the brain tissue. Certain intracranial hemorrhages, usually those large enough to cause a complete cerebral herniation or cerebral compression that is symptomatic, that is, causing a coma, a neurologic deficit, or intracranial hypertension, need to be surgically removed immediately [10].

If the initial and subsequent management of patients with TBI is not done well, patient may succumb to their injuries or end up with severe negative long-term complications. Patients with TBI have been reported to have reduced life expectancy by at least 9 years. Some of the long-term negative complications may include premature deaths resulting from seizures, accidental falls, drug poisoning, infections such as pneumonia, frequent hospitalization, high dependence on others for support in activities of daily living (ADLs), increased use of illicit brews, and moderate or severe disabilities. Other complications include impaired physical abilities, cognitive impairments such as memory loss, attention deficit, altered behavior and personality that may present through lethargy, depression, temper tantrums, and communication difficulties due to speech impairments.

8. Conclusion

Treating patients with severe TBI is still a challenge. Studies have significantly contributed in understanding the mechanism of injury and general hospital care. There is need for more studies to support in establishment of evidence-based therapeutic approaches to reduce variations in patient management and improve functional outcomes.

Author details

Pauline N. Kariuki[1*] and Motari Omariba[2]

1 Department of Nursing, Mong'oni Dispensary, Masaba North Sub-County, Nyamira County, Keroka, Kenya

2 Department of Physiotherapy, Kenya Medical Training College (KMTC), Homa Bay, Kenya

*Address all correspondence to: pnjoki2019@gmail.com

References

[1] Hyder AA, Wunderlich CA, Puvanachandra P, Gururaj G, Kobusingye OC. The impact of traumatic brain injuries: A global perspective. NeuroRehabilitation. 2007;**22**:341-353

[2] Centers for Disease Control and Prevention. National Center for Injury Prevention and Control. Web-Based Injury Statistics Query and Reporting System (WISQARS). 2005. Available from: https://www.cdc.gov/injury/wisqars [Accessed: January 29, 2024]

[3] Raskin S, Mateer C, editors. Neuropsychological Management of Mild Traumatic Brain Injury. New York: Oxford University Press; 2000

[4] Taylor CA, Bell JM, Breiding MJ, Xu L. Traumatic brain injury-related emergency department visits, hospitalizations, and deaths—United States, 2007 and 2013. MMWR Surveillance Summaries. 2017;**66**(9):1-16. DOI: 10.15585/mmwr.ss6609a1

[5] Dikmen SS, Machamer JE, Powell JM, Temkin NR. Outcome 3 to 5 years after moderate to severe traumatic brain injury. Archives of Physical Medicine and Rehabilitation. 2003;**84**(10):1449-1457. DOI: 10.1016/S0003-9993(03)00287-9

[6] Maas AI, Stocchetti N, Bullock R. Moderate and severe traumatic brain injury in adults. Lancet Neurology. 2008;7(8):728-741. DOI: 10.1016/S1474-4422(08)70164-9

[7] Nelson LD, LaRoche AA, Pfaller AY, et al. Prospective, head-to-head study of three computerized neurocognitive assessment tools (CNTs): Reliability and validity for the assessment of sport-related concussion. Journal of the International Neuropsychological Society. 2016;**22**(1):24-37. DOI: 10.1017/S1355617715001101

[8] Nelson LD, Furger RE, Ranson J, et al. Acute clinical predictors of symptom recovery in emergency department patients with uncomplicated mild traumatic brain injury (mTBI) or non-mTBI injuries. Journal of Neurotrauma. 2018;**35**(2):249-259. DOI: 10.1089/neu.2017.4988

[9] Dikmen S, Machamer J, Temkin N. Mild traumatic brain injury: Longitudinal study of cognition, functional status, and post-traumatic symptoms. Journal of Neurotrauma. 2017;**34**(8):1524-1530. DOI: 10.1089/neu.2016.4618

[10] Teasdale G, Jennett B. Assessment of coma and impaired consciousness: A practical scale. Lancet. 1974;**2**(7872):81-84

[11] Bruns J, Hauser WA. The epidemiology of traumatic brain injury: A review. Epilepsia. 2003;**44**:2-10. DOI: 10.1046/j.1528-1157.44.s10.3.x

[12] Andriessen TM, Jacobs B, Vos PE. Clinical characteristics and pathophysiological mechanisms of focal and diffuse traumatic brain injury. Journal of Cellular and Molecular Medicine. 2010;**14**:2381-2392. DOI: 10.1111/j.1582-4934.2020.01164.x

[13] Black KL, Hanks RA, Wood DL, Zafonte RD, Cullen N, Cifu DX, et al. Blunt versus penetrating violent traumatic brain injury: Frequency and factors associated with secondary conditions and complications. The Journal of Head Trauma Rehabilitation. 2002;**17**:489-496. DOI: 10.1097/00001199-200212000-00001

[14] Warden D. Military TBI during the Iraq and Afghanistan wars. The Journal of Head Trauma Rehabilitation. 2006;**21**:398-402. DOI: 10.1097/00001199-200609000-00004

[15] Ling GS, Ecklund JM. Traumatic brain injury in modern war. Current Opinion in Anaesthesiology. 2011;**24**:124-130. DOI: 10.1097/ACO.0b013e32834458da

[16] Risdall JE, Menon DK. Traumatic brain injury. Philosophical Transactions of the Royal Society of London. Series B, Biological Sciences. 2011;**366**:241-250. DOI: 10.1098/rstb.2010.0230

[17] Skandsen T, Kvistad KA, Solheim O, Strand IH, Folvik M, Vik A. Prevalence and impact of diffuse axonal injury in patients with moderate and severe head injury: A cohort study of early magnet resonance imaging findings and 1-year outcome. Journal of Neurosurgery. 2010;**113**:556-563. DOI: 10.3171/2009.9.JNS09626

[18] Schmidt OI, Infanger M, Heyde CE, Ertel W, Stahel PF. The role of neuroinflammation in traumatic brain injury. European Journal of Trauma. 2004;**30**:135-149. DOI: 10.1007/s00068-004-1394-9

[19] Smith DH, Meaney DF, Shull WH. Diffuse axonal injuryin head trauma. The Journal of Head Trauma Rehabilitation. 2003;**18**:307-316. DOI: 10.1097/00001199-200307000-00003

[20] Ray SK, Dixon CE, Banik NL. Molecular mechanisms in the pathogenesis of traumatic brain injury. Histology and Histopathology. 2002;**17**:1137-1152. DOI: 10.14670/HH-17.1137

[21] Teasdale G, Jennett B. Assessment and prognosis of coma after head injury. Acta Neurochirurgica. 1976;**34**(1-4):45-55. DOI: 10.1007/BF01405862

[22] Davanzo J, Sieg E, Timmons S. Management of traumatic brain injury. Surgical Clinics of North America. 2017;**97**(6):1237-1253. DOI: 10.1016/j.suc.2017.08.001

[23] Watridge CB, Muhlbauer MS, Lowery RD. Traumatic carotid artery dissection: Diagnosis and treatment. Journal of Neurosurgery. 1989;**71**(6):854-857

[24] Biffl WL, Moore EE, Ryu RK, et al. The unrecognized epidemic of blunt carotid arterial injuries: Early diagnosis improves neurologic outcome. Annals of Surgery. 1998;**228**(4):462-470

[25] Miller PR, Fabian TC, Bee TK. Blunt cerebrovascular injuries: Diagnosis and treatment. The Journal of Trauma. 2001;**51**(2):279-285

[26] Oxford University Press. Oxford English Dictionary. Oxford: Oxford University Press; 2022

[27] Wolf JA, Koch PF. Disruption of network synchrony and cognitive dysfunction after traumatic brain injury. Frontiers in Systems Neuroscience. 2016;**43**:1-14

[28] Lennon MJ, Brooker H, Creese B, Thayanandan T, Rigney G, Aarsland D, et al. Lifetime traumatic brain injury and cognitive domain deficits in late time: The PROTECT-TBI cohort study. Journal of Neurotrauma. 2023;**7**:1423-1435. DOI: 10.1089/neu.2022.0360

[29] Dahm J, Ponsford J. Comparison of long-term outcomes following traumatic injury: What is the unique experience for those with brain injury compared

with orthopaedic injury? Injury. 2015;**46**(1):142-149

[30] American College of Surgeons Trauma Quality Improvement Program (ACS TQIP). Best practices in the management of traumatic brain injury. In: Feliciano D, Mattox K, Moore E, editors. Trauma. 6th ed. New York: McGraw-Hill Professional; 2008

[31] Dash H, Chavali S. Management of traumatic brain injury patients. Korean Journal of Anaesthiology. 2018;**71**(1):12-21

[32] Dash HH. Prehospital care of head injured patients. Neurology India. 2008;**56**:415-419

[33] Chesnut RM, Marshall LF, Klauber MR, Blunt BA, Baldwin N, Eisenberg HM, et al. The role of secondary brain injury in determining outcome from severe head injury. The Journal of Trauma. 1993;**34**:216-222

[34] Wijdicks EF, Bamlet WR, Maramattom BV, Manno EM, McClelland RL. Validation of a new coma scale: The FOUR score. Annals of Neurology. 2005;**58**:585-593

[35] Davis DP. Prehospital intubation of brain-injured patients. Current Opinion in Critical Care. 2008;**14**:142-148

[36] Bhalla T, Dewhirst E, Sawardekar A, Dairo O, Tobias JD. Perioperative management of the pediatric patient with traumatic brain injury. Paediatric Anaesthesia. 2012;**22**:627-640

[37] Fontanilla L. Dopamine raises ICP. Critical Care. 2001;**5**:73300

[38] Chou A, Krukowski K, Jopson T, Zhu PJ, Costa-Mattioli M, Walter P, et al. Inhibition of the integrated stress response reverses cognitive deficits after traumatic brain injury. Proceedings of the National Academy of Sciences of the United States of America. 2017;**114**:E6420-E6426

[39] Oddo M, Crippa IA, Mehta S, Menon D, Payen JF, Taccone FS, et al. Optimizing sedation in patients with acute brain injury. Critical Care. 2016;**20**:128

[40] Balestreri M, Czosnyka M, Hutchinson P, Steiner LA, Hiler M, Smielewski P, et al. Impact of intracranial pressure and cerebral perfusion pressure on severe disability and mortality after head injury. Neurocritical Care. 2006;**4**:8-13

[41] Nathens AB, Cryer HG, Fildes J. The American College of Surgeons trauma quality improvement program. The Surgical Clinics of North America. 2012;**92**:441-454

[42] Cottenceau V, Masson F, Mahamid E, Petit L, Shik V, Sztark F, et al. Comparison of effects of equiosmolar doses of mannitol and hypertonic saline on cerebral blood flow and metabolism in traumatic brain injury. Journal of Neurotrauma. 2011;**28**:2003-2012

[43] Murr R, Schürer L. Correlation of jugular venous oxygen saturation to spontaneous fluctuations of cerebral perfusion pressure in patients with severe head injury. Neurological Research. 1995;**17**:329-333

[44] Temkin NR, Dikmen SS, Wilensky AJ, Keihm J, Chabal S, Winn HR. A randomized, double-blind study of phenytoin for the prevention of post-traumatic seizures. The New England Journal of Medicine. 1990;**323**:497-502

[45] Sadaka F, Veremakis C. Therapeutic hypothermia for the management of

intracranial hypertension in severe traumatic brain injury: A systematic review. Brain Injury. 2012;**26**:899-908

[46] Shi J, Dong B, Mao Y, Guan W, Cao J, Zhu R. Review: Traumatic brain injury and hyperglycemia, a potentially modifiable risk factor. Oncotarget. 2016;**7**:71052-71061

[47] Rebuck JA, Murry KR, Rhoney DH, Michael DB, Coplin WM. Infection related to intracranial pressure monitors in adults: Analysis of risk factors and antibiotic prophylaxis. Journal of Neurology, Neurosurgery, and Psychiatry. 2000;**69**:381-384

Chapter 3

Perspective Chapter: Bambi Trauma – Surviving TBI Twice

Leslie Griffin

Abstract

This essay tells you about my two experiences with traumatic brain injury. In 1993, a woman drove into me from behind as I was walking across the street (with the walk sign!). I had two brain surgeries, and was not expected to live or work again. I did. By 2016 I was a chaired professor of law. Then a young stranger attacked me, throwing me to the ground and leaving me bleeding from my head on the street. I survived that attempted murder. I am still a law professor, teaching, writing, and thinking. This essay tells you about the attacks and my recoveries, and how I learned to take care of my brain.

Keywords: intracranial hemorrhage, hematoma, trauma, left epidural hematoma intracranially, right temporal intraparenchymal hemorrhage, recovery, time, patient, patience, assault

1. Introduction

I woke up in a hospital in Houston, Texas. I could hear some news about the presidential election on TV or from people talking about it in the hospital. It was November 2016. Why was I in Houston, as my home was in Nevada? Medical personnel and my brother told me a stranger had attacked me in Nevada. He threw me to the ground and told people there I was dying. I was in Houston to get the best medical care I could, at a hospital that specializes in brain injury.

2. The beginning

Bambi Trauma. That's what they called me at the Las Vegas hospital where, on October 7, 2016, I was delivered after a stranger threw me to the ground and left me bleeding from my head on the sidewalk. It was an otherwise-peaceful Friday afternoon in Henderson, Nevada. The paramedics took me to the hospital; the police took my attacker to jail. Today, in 2024, I still do not know why I did not have my wallet on me, as I usually carry it with me. It took everyone a few days to find me.

My records tell you a story that I cannot remember. I've paged through the detailed records that the hospital gave me. I'm a good lawyer, and teach in a law school, so I always have records of everything. I am Bambi Trauma on the forms at the beginning, as no one knew who I was. Several things stand out to me. I was the victim of "assault," suffering from "closed head injury" and "respiratory failure" [1]. I understand the first, as I was thrown on my head. But it is interesting to see how much work they had to do to keep me breathing. I was intubated at the scene of the accident as I could not breathe there. Apparently I suffered from "dyspnea," or shortness of breath. My files report a "tracheostomy tube" I learned online that a "tracheostomy is an opening created at the front of the neck so a tube can be inserted into the windpipe (trachea) to help you breathe" [2]. Tracheostomy is the hole and tracheotomy is the surgery. I also had to look up the word "atelectasis," which is the "collapse of a lung or part of a lung," as it is listed I had that [3]. I also had a feeding tube.

I noticed a few times in my files the words "intracranial hemorrhage," which is not something you want to have on your brain. They also talk about hematomas, or bruises on the brain, which are not good either. The records say they had to do an EVD on me. What is that? An External Ventricular Drain. Physicians teach me that if your spinal fluid is not working well, your brain is not really working in the right way. Sometimes they put in an EVD to get the fluid moving. Did they really carve an inch in my head and stick a drain in? Yikes! [4]. I think that's what they did to impose a right frontal ventriculostomy catheter.

As I was leaving Nevada to go to Houston, the physicians summarized my medical experience this way:

> *P:*
>
> *Neuro: Pt initially GCS 10T, intubated by EMS prior to arrival and remained intubated until she was trached on 10/12/16. GCS has continued to improve to a max of GCS 14 trach collared. Neurosurgery followed pt initially and besides R frontal subgaleal drain placement, didn't require any other neurosurgical intervention. R Frontal ventriculostomy drain was removed 10/15. Completed > 14 doses of Keppra 500mg BID.*
>
> *C-spine: C-spine precautions always in place and cleared after MRI c-spine negative for any ligamentous injury.*
>
> *Facial Fractures: R temporal & maxillary bone fracture (non-displaced) on CT scan. ENT recommended non-surgical and for pt to remain under R ear water precautions & f/u outpatient PRN.*
>
> *CV: Was initially bradycardic- in the 40's, which EKG demonstrated sinus brady w/o any heart blocks or abnormal rhythms. That has since resolved. Hemodynamically stable during hospital stay, not requiring any pressors.*
>
> *Resp: Intubated prior to hospital arrival and had Trach placed 10/12. Had moderate R pleural effusion and atelectasis-resolved after switching Vent to APRV mode. No thoracentesis required. Has been using trach collar for more than 48 hours and tolerating well without any hypoxic events.*
>
> *GI/Nutrition: Initially was NPO. PEG placed 10/12. Tolerating tf at goal. On Dulcolax for bowel regimen.*
>
> *Hematologic: Thrombocytosis -resolved.*

MSK: No injury. Initially had flaccid RUE but has regained some strength and is now 3/5 and equal with other extremities Has been OOB with PT/OT and tolerating well.

ID: Received 1 week of Ancef, after subgaleal drain placement. No evidence of infection during hospital stay [5].

I cannot tell you anything about the month from October to November. Many other helpers have filled in the details for me. I was in Las Vegas's Sunrise Hospital, and then my family flew me to Houston, Texas, where I became a patient at the TIRR Memorial Hermann Hospital, which specializes in brain injury. The attack was October 7, 2016, and the flight to Houston was October 27. I do not remember what day I woke up in Houston. I was awake by the presidential election day, November 8, 2016. I was upset that I had not been able to vote. I was trying to figure out what I had missed as Donald Trump defeated Hillary Clinton. I am a tenured constitutional law professor, so of course the presidential election received most of my attention. I *always* tell people that when you vote for the president, you vote for the Supreme Court. I knew the Court was at stake in that election, and later events proved that it was.

That means I have not one single memory of the attack or of my comatose and near-death state in the hospital. Everyone wondered if I would survive.

I did. I went from TIRR to a Houston rehab clinic, then to a hotel on the University of Houston campus, and finally to a friend's house in Houston. I used to teach at the University of Houston, which is why everyone had chosen Houston as the place to go post-Las Vegas. They took good care of me there. I went home to Nevada on December 23.

Why did I survive and work again? I provide here some reasons why I think I did.

3. The relevant past

I was and am an independent person, with strong opinions and a lot of determination. That helped my recovery post my almost-murder. Why? You will be amazed to hear that on April 6, 1993, in Phoenix, Arizona, I was hit by a car from behind as I was a pedestrian crossing the street with the walk sign (**Figure 1**). Smash to the back of my head. I had *two* brain surgeries on consecutive days in 1993. I was in a coma for a while. All the news was bad. Many people told me that brain-damaged people could not survive, work, or function, and that they had to live permanently in rehab. Some of my rehab associates told me that I should stay in Phoenix for long-term rehabilitation.

I did not. My terrific surgeon, Dr. Arnold B. Calica, wrote a letter about me on April 20, 1993, explaining I "underwent two craniotomies within 48 hours after being struck by an automobile. Her life was in serious danger, and her condition was critical" [6]. Even reading the records today, 30 years later, my medical picture appears grim. The documents record my "left epidural hematoma intracranially" and my "right temporal intraparenchymal hemorrhage" [7]. Other reports said: "She did have loss of consciousness and was reportedly combative. She has remained somewhat inappropriate since that time" [8]. One word I saw a lot in reviewing my day-to-day medical records was ... headache! I apparently had a lot of headaches, which is unsurprising after two brain surgeries. Tests showed a lot of deficits with memory and reasoning problems. I went to in-hospital rehab on April 12, when "cognitive dysfunction was present" [9]. They sent me off to the non-hospital rehab center on April 23rd.

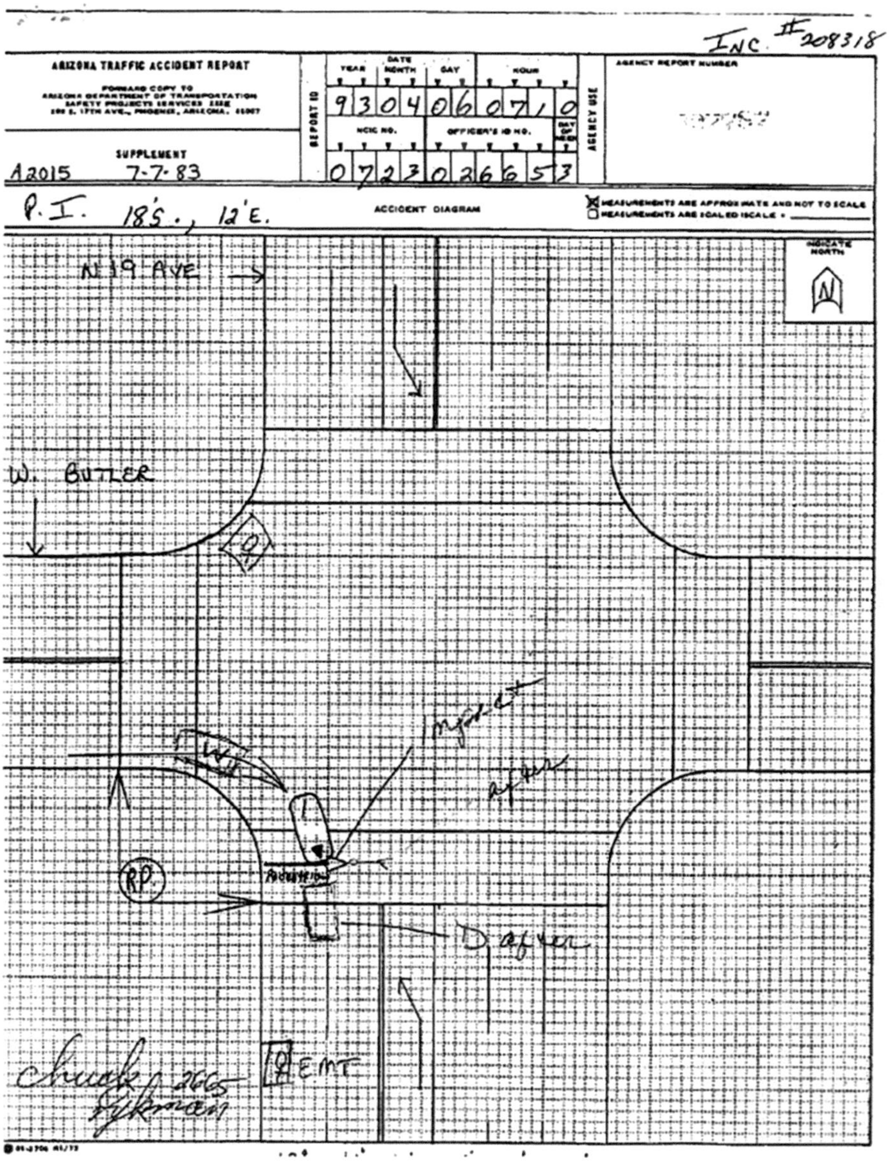

Figure 1.
That's what it looks like to be hit by a car!.

I burst out laughing when I read the chart from April 13, 1993. "Nursing states pt awoke during middle of night last pm wanting a snack. Requests an hs-snack. One is being set up" [10] Why did I laugh? Even today, when I am hungry, I want food immediately. No delay acceptable. Without food I get completely cranky. True in 1993, true in 2024! Later, on April 16, I rejected the hospital's worksheets, saying they were "silly" and that I was "too tired to participate" [11]. That sounds like me too. I apparently complained "I'm being held against my will" [11].

At first rehab review, "[i]t was determined on her psychometric evaluation, she was having a wide variety of neurocognitive memory and attentional deficits with visual spatial and frontal areas impaired. Her overall intellectual function was thought to have probably dropped and that was specifically in the performance area, visual spatial areas and verbal cognitive areas" [12].

I spent April 23–30, 1993 at one rehab hospital. After that, I visited the Adult Day Center at Barrow Neurological Institute from May 3 to May 14 [13]. At Barrow they noted "deficits in the area of visual perception and executive functioning. There were also some indications of memory deficits" [13]. My medical history shows problems with the Wisconsin Card Sorting Test. After that, I was not so good on the Booklet Category Test and the Oral Symbol Digit Test, the Trail Making Test, and the Tactile Performance Test. I suffered "moderate impairment" [13]. "They noted there are still a number of areas which are significantly below her premorbid abilities. These include delayed visual recall, overall speed of information processing, tactile perception, psychomotor tracking and simple motor speed" [13].

I observe in the reports that my communication was above average, and I had high reading comprehension. On those issues, I had a "superior level of functioning" [13]. My picture naming, however, was slow. It remained slow in later months when I faced more tests about how well I could copy a picture. And definitely my neuromuscular tests and balance were not as good as my words skills.

That is what the papers say. I remember hating rehab, and in particular many of the neuro games we played. On one test, the staff said I was too slow, and did not use the fastest way to solve the problem. I responded that I had to consider every option slowly, as I was a law clerk who always had to see all the options. I had a different problem with the Wisconsin Card Sorting Test. They ask the patient to identify the criterion determining their movements. But the criterion always changes. I thought they should have said criteria instead of criterion. I saw that as an inconsistency and therefore did not like the test. And kept failing it. People to this day say I am much too literal and the Wisconsin test probably proves that.

Once I went to out-patient rehab I was living back in my apartment. I needed a Lifeline machine that will beep and notify people if you fall or hurt yourself. I had generous neighbors who always kept an eye on me to make sure everything was okay. I was not allowed to drive, and had to spend time going to rehab, which, let me repeat, I did not enjoy at all. The one medical issue I faced was that I developed vertigo, and went to the hospital once to check on that.

I went back to work in Judge Schroeder's office on May 17, where everyone welcomed my return and supported my recovery.

On June 3, 1993 Dr. Calica wrote a memo about my frustration with intense neuropsychiatric therapy and noted I would like to stop. He thought I could leave it, and noted I was working half days at my legal job without frustration. It is true doctors always expect frustration from a brain injury patient. You get frustrated if your brain is not working the way it used to. In a later memo, July 13, 1993, Calica told the state of California that I was capable of driving.

The rehabbers noted my hyperverbality and gave me an MMPI-2 test. They wanted to keep an eye on me because of some weaknesses in all my testing.

Today, I still have stacks of files connected to this accident. The files remind me I had lawyers who handled everything, collected all my bills, made sure everything was legally sound, checked with my insurance and the driver who hit me. The bills are enormous, and both times my insurance covered most of them. That experience is why I always want everyone to have health insurance. I had federal employee health insurance the first time and state employee insurance the second. It does pay most of your bills, which is much better than paying thousands of dollars yourself.

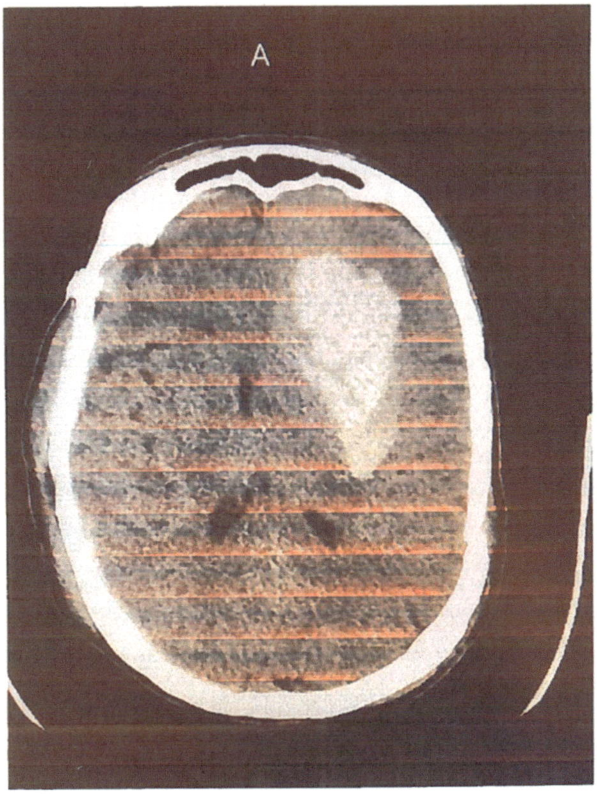

Figure 2.
My brain (1), October 2016.

I left Phoenix, and attended the Harvard fellowship I had won before the accident. I had a doctor there who had worked with a brain-injured patient and knew the patient had recovered. Her confidence in that patient added to my own growing sense that I could be okay. Neuropsychologist Dr. Dorene Rentz guided me through the ups and downs of brain recovery and stress.

For the record, the medical tests that my Nevada doctors did on me in 2016 observe that I had had two craniotomies (**Figures 2** and **3**) [14]. The effects of surgery stay on your brain! The experience of Phoenix stayed with me in Nevada. I had survived brain injury before and knew that I could do it again.

4. My characteristics

How did I survive this? First, I was almost always *cranky*. There's no way around that. In my mind, there is nothing good about being in a hospital. Nothing at all. All of it is terrible. I expressed my crankiness quite frequently.

My friends have all told me that no matter what anyone did, I was always trying to get free of the hospital, of the room, and of any restraints they placed on me. Everyone was horrified by my actions, and I think some believed it was proof of my brain damage. My attempts meant I did not have the discipline to stay put. The hospital staff closed my bedroom door, blocked the elevator, kept their eyes on me, etc.,

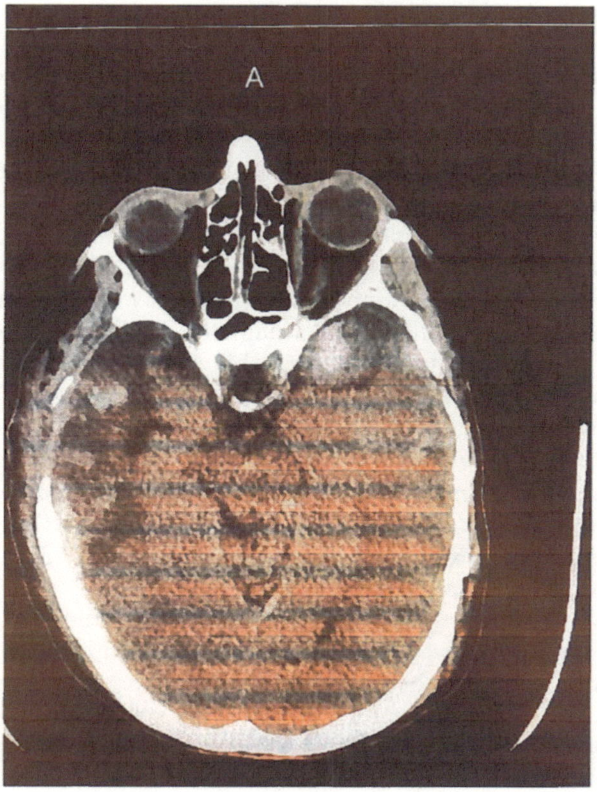

Figure 3.
My brain (2), October 2016.

etc., etc. It bothered the rest of you that all I wanted was to be free. In my mind, it is a sign of *health*. No healthy person wants to be in a hospital, and so I joined the healthy in trying to escape. I was always cranky when I could not.

My brother tells me he has a friend who works with brain patients. She warned him that once I came to, I would be horrible to deal with. He tells me that I was. I kept telling him negative things and how I did not like anything, including him. He dealt with it because she told him that being cranky is part of recovery. I am proof of that.

This *cranky* person is also *independent.* I like that word, "independent," more than the word "autonomy," a word we traditionally use in bioethics. I teach Bioethics, which is the ethics of medicine and medical research. In Fall Semester 2016 I was using the first edition of my casebook, *Practicing Bioethics Law*, to teach a seminar at the law school. So I knew a lot—academically—about patient autonomy, a term that usually means that the patient gets to hear full information from the doctor and to give her informed consent to any procedures she undergoes.

I was independent in Nevada and Texas because I had that 1993 experience in my brain and in my body. I had definitely beaten the odds in Round One. Let me emphasize, it was not *easy*. Nevertheless, from 1993 to 2016 I attended my fellowship at Harvard University, received a tenure-track position at a law school, worked in the Office of Professional Responsibility at the U.S. Department of Justice, got law-school tenure, received a chaired position at one law school, and then a chair at another school, wrote many articles and textbooks, and filed some amicus briefs in different courts of appeals. By October 2016 I was leading the good life, and not even thinking about whether I was brain damaged way back in 1993.

My attacker tried to take all that away from me in 2016, as the car driver had in 1993. Why was I independent as well as cranky? Because *no one* was going to tell me that my brain did not work. *No one. Period.* Family, friend, doctor, researcher, genius. I did not listen. I told myself they had been wrong before and now were wrong again.

Admittedly, it is *easier* the second time than the first. By then you know better than anyone what to expect, and have learned life lessons that never desert you. Brain Injury 2? I had survived Round One so I knew what I had to do.

Do you prefer the word *stubborn* or *resilient*? Allied to my independence was a stubborn commitment to my well-being, through thick and thin, good and bad. A good friend who works in medicine tells me stubborn sounds negative, and resilient is more positive. I agree. It is. But I think stubborn describes me better. Whatever happened, I stubbornly proceeded as if I were healthy and my brain was still functioning. From Injury 1, I knew that recovery would take time, so I gave it to myself. I knew recovery was not a sign of permanent damage. It was just part of the long slow process that recovery involves.

For every medical person reading this, I want you to acknowledge that recovery takes *time*. I knew that, so I waited for it. My insurers were not as patient. At the beginning of my injury, they were ready to give up on me after 2 weeks, suggesting I be sent to a permanent rehab home because the 2 weeks made it clear I was not going to heal. My insurance law colleague had to fight with them to extend their coverage. My advice? Do not watch the clock. Rehab takes *time.* Families, do not give up on your loved ones too early. Many of us are still in there, recovering, and just waiting for the opportunity to tell you how terrible the whole experience is and how glad we are to see you.

Traumatic Brain Injury also involves *sorrow.* I will not pretend that going through brain injury once or twice was fun or relaxing. I was filled with sorrow. I could not believe that I would have to prove my intellectual talents again, as I had been required to do in 1993. Then 59 years old, with my chaired professorship, would I really have to convince people I could still think? By pure coincidence I was on sabbatical in spring 2017, so I used the time to rest. I gave three talks, two that were scheduled pre-attack. At a bioethics conference, I talked about my experience of attack and injury. No one seemed to believe I was too injured to work.

Imagine going back to UNLV in Fall 2017 to teach my first law class after everyone knew about the whole trauma from reading it in the newspapers and talking about it at school. And, of course, there were all those students who had lost me halfway through the Fall 2016 semester. I kept wondering if students would quickly recognize I was brain damaged and start talking about it among themselves. That was a lot of stress. Recovery from brain injury is bound to give you stress.

Yet I kept going. But I felt incredible sorrow that I had to go through this a second time. I had strength from having learned about it the first time, but sorrow that I had to prove myself again.

I believe that my *strength* came from the first experience. I had learned once that the brain can recover. It was a lesson I knew and remembered, and I did not have to learn it again. I knew it with all my heart, soul, and mind, and that memory kept me going even when times were hard, even when everyone else was giving up on me.

Were times *hard*? Yes. In 2017, I wrote about the attack, and noted that I felt *fear* and *caution* [15]. I did and I do. I think any hospital experience of illness brings about those reactions. It is hard to live when your body has been beaten to a pulp, or to survive when you have almost died. Your body needs recovery time to get your strength back. Recovery does not come all in 1 day. It takes time for the various parts of the body to heal. Any patient knows this and may show it in fearful and cautious use of their body parts. We do not want to reinjure body parts that have already survived an attack and much illness.

I had an additional fear and caution, both times. A driver ran me over, and a stranger tried to kill me. Neither illness started in my own body. The injuries were imposed by others. Post-1993, I used to joke that you could tell me I was winning the Nobel Prize in a crosswalk and I would not hear you because my eyes were always on the traffic. Today I do not let anyone walk behind me. I live in a beautiful Nevada park. I'm sure it looks weird that I always look behind me and sometimes stop so people can pass me. Why? Because someone tried to murder me from behind. I do not remember the attempted murder, but my body is always protecting itself. Why? I think *fear* and *caution* are a normal part of the patient's life, and being an attacked patient makes them worse. I accept my fear and caution as a normal part of an attack victim's life, and never dismiss them as a weakness.

I also know that you have to respond to brain injury with *confidence.* To get through the hell of brain injury, you need to have confidence. Why? Because in my view the best thing you can do is keep your brain working, not accepting that its prime is past. You've got to believe your brain is working and keep using it to show it can work. Otherwise, it will just rest until it gets worn out from not working at all. It matters if you keep telling patients they can and should use their brains. That is much better than telling them to rest all the time, as my hospital doctors used to do. You cannot work all the time, but you can use your brain and keep it active.

I really know this lesson about confidence. In 1993, no one was confident about me. A lot of doctors told me the brain could not heal at all. Once it was hurt, they said, it was gone. They gave me tons of tests in rehab to prove that. They urged me to rehab my way through life and accept all the limitations that a car driver had imposed on me. All those negative talks influenced me in the post-1993 years. I always felt that I had to prove myself to other people. I did feel like I had to show I was not the brain-injured legal clerk who had lost her career on the streets of Phoenix. Being told you are brain damaged and cannot do anything because everyone will notice your injury does not aid your health. It is a terrible way to go through life. The negative message undermined my confidence for years. But I stubbornly kept that confidence because it was the only thing that kept me going.

For the record, I think all those brain tests proved I am not an athlete! I later learned from my athletic coach that no one can survive negative people with negative world views. Athletes take failure as a lesson, not as a reason to stop working. Many brain-injured people stop thinking because their helpers keep telling them they are brain injured and cannot get better. That discouragement takes recovery away from people. I know that because I faced it and confronted it. For the first injury, the rehabbers' negative remarks stayed with me long-term. I had to face the negative down. Fortunately, my neurosurgeon and my Massachusetts doctors were much more positive, so I kept strong in my own confidence by hearing their confidence in me and in their other patients.

5. Others

That's why every patient needs at least one *advocate*. I was lucky because I had many, through first and second injuries. My mother was still alive during the first, and my siblings during the second. They flew in to see me and to help however they could. Many people, including my colleagues and students, visited me repeatedly, keeping me company through my agony. Or, at the beginning, they told me, they just stood there hoping I would wake up and talk to them. Colleagues whose career is studying insurance and health law made sure my insurance would give me full coverage and help instead of hurt. Many friends stayed up on my down days. They did tons of work that I have completely forgotten. Pulling for me and, of course, taking over my classes when I could not teach anything.

I'll say it a million times. TBI is a terrible experience. It tests every element of you and your life. After the second attack, I thought a lot about quitting. Retiring. When someone almost takes your life away, you wonder if you should keep working. You wonder if it is not better to quit, especially as many people think you cannot work. So why try? Let me repeat what I said above. Your brain will not work if you do not use it. It's like any other part of body exercise that I learned from my coach. If you do not use it, you lose it. So TBI survivors everywhere, do not let anyone tell you to stop trying. Do not overwork your brain. But use it to keep it strong. You can retire from many things, but do not quit. Be patient with a slow recovery, but do something for your recovery every day.

I'm grateful for all the help I received from so many, family, friends, colleagues, students, nurses, doctors, and rehab experts. UNLV had to fill in for me with other professors when I could not show up, mid-semester, to do my job. And there was never any thought that they were going to fire or replace me because of my illness. That is lucky, because some TBI patients lose their jobs very quickly.

Yet you also may have to recover *alone*. Especially women. There are many studies now that show that women receive different medical treatment than men [16]. Medicine is often geared to men's bodies more than women's, and women's complaints of pain are also taken less seriously than men's [17]. I have seen studies that women patients lose caretakers more quickly than men do, and that many women lose their spouses because the husbands cannot tolerate the wives' injuries. Without a caretaker, you are alone. Women often are, as I have been. Recently I told my athletic coach what I concentrate on and what's important in my thinking of day-to-day life as someone who has recovered from brain injury. And he said, "no man would want to put up with that." It's a stark statement, but there is some truth to it. If you are focused on rehabbing your brain so that it works as it always did, you may spend a lot of time alone, just making sure your brain can work. That may not appeal to you, but it also may be a part of recovery for many women who suffer TBI.

6. Lessons learned

I wrote in such detail about my TBIs because I think it is very important for people to understand the lived experience of the *patient*'s brain injury. Dr. William Winslade was my colleague at the University of Houston Law Center, and then invited me back to the University of Texas Medical Branch (UTMB) at Galveston post-my attempted murder. Winslade has had a significant effect on bioethics and medicine. The title of his book, Confronting Traumatic Brain Injury: Devastation, Hope, and Healing, captures much of what brain injury patients go through [18]. I hope this chapter shows you how devastation, hope and healing affected me. Twice.

Like me, Winslade faced a brain injury that was supposed to kill him or ruin his life. It did not. He has lived a full and happy life. He knows, as I know, that one successful patient can help another to heal. If I can heal twice, you can heal too. Medicine needs to be full of the stories of patients who heal, not only of those who do not.

Doctors need to remember this. Sometimes doctors expect everyone to follow the same scientific experience. As they told me in Phoenix, brain damage ends your life. Period. Do not ask us about that, they said. Just know your life has changed.

In contrast, some doctors have emphasized that, while technology gives great insight into human health, medicine should never lose sight of the "physical exam and humanistic aspects of medicine. Overall, a machine cannot offer a shoulder to cry on, a warm hand to hold or words of comfort during a life-altering diagnosis" [19]. The "iPatient" [19] is never the whole patient. These doctors hope that artificial intelligence "can allow us to spend more time interacting with our patients" [19]. This is what patients look for. Doctors who understand their experience and give them hope.

I still hate to look at the brain slides I attached to this chapter. But my story should tell you I am much more than the iPatient pictures the doctors interpreted. They had to deal with me and not just with my technology.

Neuroscientist Adrian Owen explained this in his book, Into the Gray Zone. He learned that medicine involves both caring for people and scientific discovery [20].

Joseph Fins is a doctor who has taught us so much about the brain. Dr. Winslade introduced me to Dr. Fins when Fins gave one of his brilliant lectures at UTMB. Unbelievably, before Fins met me, some of my colleagues had asked him at a different conference if I would be able to recover. As a surgeon, Fins understood that patients are in different circumstances. He explained that some patients achieve a minimally conscious state that gives them the ability to communicate and relate with other people [21].

Fins emphasized that brain injury had taught him, and should teach us, that patients have a right to *care*. In law and bioethics, we frequently discuss the right to die. There are lead Supreme Court cases on death that are in the early chapters of my bioethics book. Remember Karen Ann Quinlan and Nancy Cruzan, two cases about just what rights individuals have about their deaths and how to manage them? [22].

Dr. Fins says brain injury should teach people to care for our patients, who are all in different circumstances, not just about their deaths. He invited me to talk about Neurorehabilitation and Society: Going through Hell, at the 2022 International Neuroethics Meeting. His important book has another inspirational title: Rights Come to Mind: Brain Injury, Ethics, and the Struggle for Consciousness [23]. Rights. That's what bioethics is supposed to support. Patients' rights to live and be healthy. My insurance company, you learned above, was ready to give up on me too early. Patients need care and attention, and it usually takes time and patience for them to heal.

As I've tried to explain in my story, brain injury patients are often ignored, told they cannot live well and that they cannot recover. Fins's awareness of the treatment of brain-injured patients made him a member of the community of advocates for the disabled. In one article, he joins a group of scholars explaining that the Americans With Disabilities Act has not done enough to integrate the disabled into society. These authors propose instead an Americans With Abilities Act. They identify different ways the law can help people live lives of ability. They explain how their statute will work "*prospectively* through the provision of technologies that help individuals achieve their forward-looking potential" [24].

Abilities, even in the saddest circumstances. Their message is positive. As the message must be if patients are to recover. It was the positive, pro-future people who always helped me.

As a last note, I rarely talk about any books or articles on insurance. I know people who do not believe in health insurance, or do not want to pay anything for it. I have a very strong message on this, and it does not rely on anything I've read. I tell people you never know when one—or two—days may require you to pay a lot of health bills for injury to your brain. Be sure to get insurance so that if TBI happens to you, you will not have to pay thousands and thousands of dollars in bills.

7. Conclusion

I hope you never have to join me on the recovery road. For those of you who do, stay positive. You can do it. With the help of your medical personnel, who should know they should always send you a positive message that you can do well. That you can use your brain and build your future.

But remember it is *your* brain, not mine. Mine is good at communication and writing, which are academic skills. Today it just amuses me that my athletic and other talents are not as good. I can accept that. I am happy I am still working. The rest of you may have different talents. Do what your brain allows you to do.

The brain is remarkable. So be sure to use yours.

Acknowledgments, notes and thanks

Many people saw me through these traumas. My late mother, Doris Schanning Griffin, my sister Deborah Griffin, and my brother Joe Griffin. Dr. Arnold Calica was a fabulous surgeon who helped me get back to my clerkship with the wonderful Judge Mary Murphy Schroeder in Phoenix. Dr. Dorene Rentz helped cure me from the first accident. Kevin Worth supported all my efforts to heal. Ruben Garcia and Tori Carreon helped find me in the Las Vegas hospital after I did not show up for a Friday night dinner. Stacey Tovino is a great health and insurance lawyer. Joan Krause is also a health care lawyer who paid my bills and kept her eyes on things while I was unconscious. Darlene Walker visited me in the Houston hospitals and took me into her home post-discharge. Nadine Matta Balombin offered steady care. Vegas's Nancy Rapoport, Whitney Short, and Erica Medley kept me focused on recovery, and made sure my legal papers were in order. Dr. William Winslade and Dr. Joseph Fins gave me great insight into the brain and encouraged me to write about it. And there are many, many more, to whom I send my thanks.

Conflict of interest

The author declares no conflict of interest.

Author details

Leslie Griffin
University of Nevada, Las Vegas, USA

*Address all correspondence to: leslie.griffin@unlv.edu

References

[1] Patient: Trauma, Bambi, and then Griffin, Leslie, Sunset Hospital, Las Vegas, NV. 2016

[2] Overview: Tracheostomy. NHS. 2019. Available from: https://www.nhs.uk/conditions/tracheostomy/#:~:text=A%20tracheostomy%20is%20an%20opening,breathing%20machine%20called%20a%20ventilator

[3] Atelectasis Overview. MayoClinic. Available from: https://www.mayoclinic.org/diseases-conditions/atelectasis/symptoms-causes/syc-20369684

[4] Cleveland Clinic. External Ventricular Drain (EVD). 2020. Available from: https://www.youtube.com/watch?v=Tul9sm30QNo

[5] Patient: Griffin, Leslie. Sunrise Hospital, Las Vegas, NV. 2016

[6] Calica AB. Letter to Relatives of Leslie Griffin. 1993

[7] John C. Lincoln Hospital & Health Center. X-Ray Consultation. Griffin, Leslie. p. 2

[8] John C. Lincoln Hospital & Health Center. Critical Care Consultation Report. 1993

[9] John C. Lincoln Hospital. Discharge Summary. Griffin, Leslie. 1993

[10] Lincoln Patient Progress Note. April 13, 1993

[11] Lincoln Patient Progress Note. April 16, 1993

[12] John C. Lincoln Hospital & Health Center. Admit for Rehabilitation. 1993

[13] Barrow Neurological Institute. Initial Program Summary. 1993

[14] Patient: Trauma, Bambi. Sunrise Hospital, Las Vegas, NV. 2016

[15] Griffin LC. Pre- or post-mortem? Nevada Law Journal. 2017;**18**:221-227

[16] Gordon D. Almost 50% of young women report negative healthcare experiences, new study shows. Forbes. 24 Feb 2023. Available from: https://www.forbes.com/sites/debgordon/2023/02/24/almost-50-of-young-women-report-negative-healthcare-experiences-new-study-shows/

[17] Chen PG et al. Gender Differences in Patients' Experience of Care in the Emergency Department. 37 Concise Research Report2002. pp. 676-679

[18] Winslade W. Confronting Traumatic Brain Injury: Devastation, Hope and Healing. New Haven, CT: Yale University Press; 1998

[19] Balancing Technology and Human Connection in Patient Care. Stanford Medicine. 2023. Available from: https://stanfordmedicine25.stanford.edu/blog/archive/2023/significanceofsmallgestures1.html

[20] Owen A. Into the Gray Zone: A Neuroscientist Explores the Border between Life and Death. New York: Scribner; 2017

[21] Fins JJ. Brain injury: Neuroscience and Neuroethics. Hastings Center Bioethics Briefing. 21 Sep 2015. Available from: https://www.thehastingscenter.org/briefingbook/the-vegetative-and-minimally-conscious-states/

[22] In the Matter of Karen Quinlan, 355 A.2d 647. 1976; Cruzan v. Missouri Department of Health, 497 U.S. 261. 1990

[23] Fins JJ. Rights Come to Mind: Brain Injury, Ethics, and the Struggle for Consciousness. Cambridge: Cambridge University Press; 2015

[24] Fins JJ et al. Designing an Americans with abilities act: Consciousness, capabilities, and civil rights. Boston College Law Review. 1729;**2022**(63): 1729-1796

Chapter 4

Brain Concussion: Recent Advances, Outcomes, and Challenges

Ahmad Tamimi, Iskandar Tamimi, Mohamad Barbarawi, Abdel Karim Qudah and Faleh Tamimi

Abstract

The concept of brain concussion is still controversial among researchers and clinicians who address this type of head injury from different perspectives. Some clinicians prefer the term "concussion," while others favor the term "mild traumatic brain injury" (mTBI). Brain concussion, or mild head injury, affects temporary brain function with clinical symptoms that may include loss of consciousness, memory loss, blurred vision, and confusion. The main etiology includes road traffic accidents, falls, and sports injuries. Brain concussion, or mTBI, is the most common type of head injury. The definition and pathophysiology of this condition are still controversial since research on this topic has been mainly based on animal experimentation. However, recent advances, including neuroimages and neurophysiology, have improved the understanding of brain concussion. This chapter will address the history, background, definition, classification, diagnosis, symptoms, complications, outcome, treatment, prevention, and challenges related to this condition.

Keywords: brain concussion, mild traumatic brain injury, post-concussion syndrome, sports medicine, outcome

1. Introduction

1.1 History of brain concussion

The Hippocratic Corpus, a collection of ancient Greek texts written in the fifth and fourth centuries BCE, used for the first time the term concussion (**Figure 1**). This term was later translated to "commotion cerebri" and included the loss of speech, hearing, and sight that could result from a "commotion of the brain" [1]. Hippocratic Corpus mentioned concussion.

Muhammad Ibn Zakariya Razi was the first to differentiate between brain concussions and other types of head injuries in the tenth century [2]. He is also believed to have been the first to adopt the term "cerebral concussion." In his definition of brain

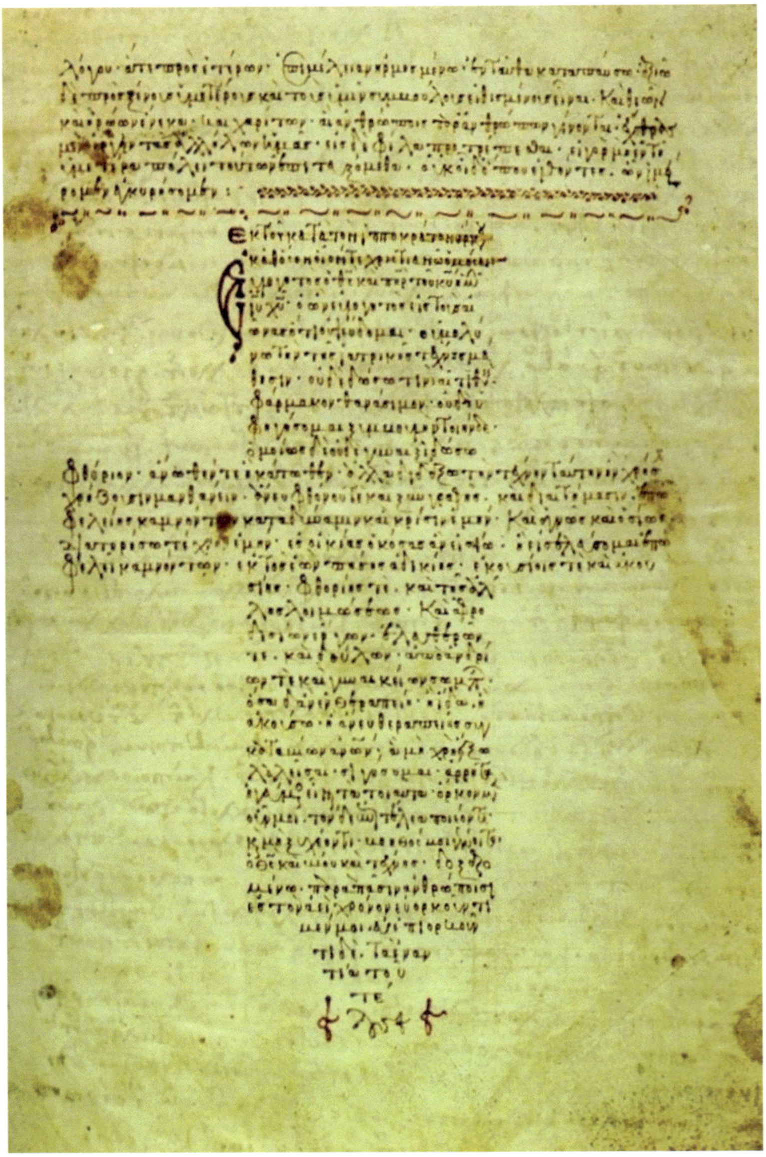

Figure 1.
The Hippocratic Corpus mentioned brain concussion.

concussion, he included a transient loss of function in the absence of physical damage, which set the basis for the understanding of this entity in the coming centuries [3].

Lanfrancus in the thirteenth century expanded this concept of brain concussion as brain commotion and described the difference between concussion and other types of head injuries. And described the post-concussion symptoms as a consequence of the transient loss of consciousness [4]. In the fourteenth century, Guy de Chauliac described the relatively good outcome of brain concussion. In the sixteenth century, the term concussion was used for symptoms such as confusion, lethargy, and memory problems [4]. Ambroise Pare used the term "shaking brain" for brain concussion [1]. In 1839, Dupuytren Guillaume differentiated between brain contusion, which was considered a head injury associated with brain damage, and brain concussion, which was not associated with brain damage [4]. In 1940, animal experiments showed no microscopic damage after brain concussions [5].

1.2 The terminology of brain concussion

The World Health Organization's (WHO) Collaborating Centre Task Force on Mild Traumatic Brain Injury has observed that there are 38 definitions used in literature to define brain concussion, as well as numerous terminologies (i.e., mild Traumatic Brain Injury (mTBI), minor TBI, concussion, etc.) [6].

The most common (TBI) severity classification is the Glasgow Coma Scale (GCS), which ranges from 13 to 15 for brain concussion. However, infants, young children, and patients with pre-existing neurological disorders are difficult to assess using this scale [7].

Accordingly, mTBI is defined by a 30-minute post-trauma GCS score between 13 and 15, in addition to one or more of the following: <30 minute loss of consciousness; <24 hour impaired mental state; confusion or disorientation at the time of the accident; and transient neurological deficit. Some authors prefer to use the term "complicated mild TBI" in patients with visible lesions on the (Computerized Tomography) CT scan and/or MRI. Whereas, other researchers suggest that these cases should be defined as "moderate TBI" [8].

Concussion has been defined as a complex pathophysiological process as a result of head trauma, which leads to a series of non-specific signs or symptoms and/or changes in mental function [9].

Concerning the American Association of Neurosurgery (AANS), the definition of brain concussion is an injury to the brain that results in temporary loss of normal brain function. Medically, it is defined as a clinical syndrome characterized by an immediate and transient alteration in brain function, including an alteration in the mental status, or level of consciousness, that results from the mechanical force of the initial trauma [10]. Mild traumatic brain injuries have a temporal effect on brain function [11]. causing loss of consciousness, memory loss, headache, difficulty in thinking and concentration, blurring of vision, and mood changes [12]. These symptoms may appear immediately or days after the injury. In the case of sport-related concussions, 10% may be associated with loss of consciousness [12].

2. The epidemiology of brain concussion

The prevalence of mTBI is difficult to measure; some authors have found that up to 36.4% of the population may experience at least one mTBI during their lifetime [13]. The overall incidence rate of TBI in the US for 2002–2006 was 579 per 100,000 inhabitants [14]. However, these numbers include all TBI of different severities. Moreover, the hospitalization rate related to TBI in the US was 93.8 per 100,000 inhabitants. In a meta-analysis that reviewed TBIs from different European countries from the 1990s and the 2000s, it observed a TBI rate of 235 per 100,000 inhabitants [15, 16].

The vast majority of TBIs (up to 90%) are classified as "mild" (mTBI) [17]. The incidence of mTBI has been reported to range between 200 and 300 and 100,000 persons per year for hospitalized patients and probably twice as high if non-hospitalized patients are included. However, a few recent population-based studies reported a much higher rate (>700/100,000) [18].

There is a significant variation in the incidence of head injuries depending on the sport and age of the athletes. Moreover, many head injuries are underreported due to their mild nature and sometimes due to the fear of medical disqualification [19]. The incidence of mTBI in high school athletes is 0.59/1000 males (i.e., this incidence is almost twice as high in females), and it accounts for 15% of all sport-related injuries in high school athletes [20]. It is estimated that in the USA it may range between 1.4 and 3.8 million cases per year [21]. The annual prevalence of Canadians reporting a concussion was 110 per 100,000 population; it was more likely to affect younger males, mainly between the ages of 16 and 34. And more than 54% of all concussions were sport-related [22].

A changing pattern in the epidemiology of TBI has been found in high-income countries, related to a decrease in the incidence of road traffic accident-related injuries, especially in young adults. In contrast, these injuries have become more common in the elderly population as a result of accidental falls [18].

3. Etiology of brain concussion

A concussion occurs as a result of direct or indirect force. The head trauma can lead to an acute acceleration-deceleration injury to the brain, which consequently leads to a concussion [23]. As mentioned above, common causes of brain concussion include road traffic accidents (RTAs), falls, sports injuries, and bicycle accidents [24]. Risky factors may include alcohol, physical violence, and a prior history of concussion [25]. Elderly patients and children under the age of 4 years are also at a greater risk of suffering concussions. TBIs are commonly caused by bicycle falls in adolescents and exposure to explosive devices in military staff [26]. In athletes, the risk for concussion is greatest in American football, rugby, hockey, and soccer players, respectively. In young women and girls, the risk is greatest in soccer and basketball. An athlete who has a history of one or more concussions is at greater risk of being diagnosed with another concussion [27].

3.1 Sport: Brain concussion

The risk of injury is inherent to the practice of sports. This risk depends on the nature of the game and the specific activities of the participants. For example, American football and ice hockey are known to result in more acute traumatic injuries than other sports, and boxing is associated with a high number of head-related traumas. Each sport may have specific types of injuries, some of which could be unique to the sport. However, brain concussions may occur in any sport or physical activity. Accordingly, the number of collisions in a practice or game is directly related to the potential for concussion [28], which is the most common type of acute brain injury in sports. Accordingly, brain concussion is most frequently associated with ice hockey, boxing, American football, and martial arts [29].

Research has shown that up to 20% of high school football injuries were brain concussions. Moreover, up to 14% of the high school football players reported to have experienced at least one episode of concussion with loss of consciousness [30].

In another study, the brain concussion rate (i.e., per 100 player seasons) was found to be 1.14 for female soccer, 0.92 for male soccer, 3.66 for American football, 1.58 for wrestling, 0.46 for softball, 0.23 for baseball, 1.04 for female basketball, 0.75 for male basketball, 0.46 for field hockey, and 0.14 for volleyball. The median time lost after a brain concussion was 3 days, and 76.1% of the athletes missed <8 days. Brain concussion rates were overall higher in games than in practice, except in the case of volleyball. [31].

Some brain concussion monitoring programs have been described to reduce its frequency through ongoing surveillance programs [32]. Any program must emphasize the prevention of brain concussions by focusing on the rules and regulations of the different sports. In addition, the coaches must be trained with the appropriate skills to guarantee the safety of the players.

The assessment of sport-related injury patterns has evolved significantly over time in order to improve safety and to create accurate prevention programs. For example, Haddon's model includes 3-time phases, which include variables associated with the athlete, sport, and environment [33]. The early identification of brain concussions is essential to provide adequate management of these injuries, reduces the risk of potential negative outcomes, and increases the probability of returning to competition without exposing the athlete to a high risk of re-injury. The follow-up of brain concussions should include athlete-reported symptoms, potential signs of incomplete recovery, and protocols to assess the neuropsychological function of the brain.

3.2 Military: Brain concussion

Brain concussion is the most common traumatic brain injury affecting military personnel [34]. The prevalence of mTBI among returning service members ranges from 15.2% to 22.8% [35]. In combat zones, the majority of brain concussions result from blunt traumatisms from explosive devices [36]. Moreover, approximately 10–15% of patients may develop long-term symptoms or post-concussive syndrome (PCS). The signs and symptoms of PCS may include irritability, sleeping disorders, memory loss, anxiety, headaches, and concentration problems [37].

A blast injury results in blast winds, a rapid acoustic wave that passes through the brain tissue [38]. Approximately 80% of all the traumatic brain injuries resulting from blasts are brain concussions [39]. The degree of the damage that results from the blast depends on many factors, such as the explosive type, distance, its occurrence in an open or closed space, and the presence of interposing solid structures. The reflection of the blast waves on different surfaces can result in multiple pressure waves, which may continue to impact the victim from different angles after the initial blast [40].

Military-related concussions are difficult to evaluate and may vary significantly in severity. Moreover, there are still no validated biomarkers for the assessment of these injuries. Acute blast-related brain concussions are characterized by multifocal axonal injury, neural inflammation, vascular damage, and high p-tau levels. These changes are generally reversible and usually improve with rest. However, there are no well-established tools to follow up on the status of these patients or to predict their prognosis.

3.3 RTA and falls and brain concussion

The two most common causes of traumatic brain injury are falls and RTAs, which include vehicle collisions, car-motorcycle collisions, pedestrians run over by a vehicle, vehicle-cyclist accidents, and bicycle and motorcycle accidents. Road traffic accidents have been traditionally considered to be the most common cause of traumatic brain injury. However, a study published in 2013 reported that falls are now the leading cause of traumatic head injury [41].

3.4 Shaken baby syndrome

It is considered to be a type of physical child abuse, which is defined as the manual shaking of an infant who is being held by the extremities or shoulders, leading to whiplash-induced intracranial and intraocular bleeding and no external signs of head trauma. [42]. The majority of the victims are between 3 and 8 months of age. However, shaken baby syndrome may occur in children up to 5 years of age [43]. A rotational acceleration and deceleration force on the infant's head cause the brain to rotate in the skull. Causing retinal hemorrhages, which are frequently extensive and may extend to through the layers of the retina and much of the circumference of the globe [44, 45]. In a neuropathological study, hypoxic–ischemic findings were detected rather than the diffuse axonal injury usually seen in older children and adults with fatal head trauma [46].

4. Biomechanics of brain concussion

It is broadly defined as the interrelation between the forces experienced during the impact, the head and neck movements, and the stiffness of the tissues that compose the head/neck complex. The deformation of structures at the macroscopic and microscopic level, and the biological responses to the various loading conditions imposed on the head. The biological responses may be structural (torn vessels and axons) or functional (changes in blood flow or neurological status), and they may be immediate or delayed.

A good understanding of the biomechanics of brain concussions in children is essential to designing specific protective devices for this age group. In addition, this understanding would aid sports experts in creating sport-specific rules aimed at reducing the risk of brain concussion in children. [42].

5. Pathophysiology

After a brain concussion, a complex set of processes occurs that disrupt neuronal functioning and result in different signs and symptoms [47]. Immediately after a traumatic event to the brain, the acceleration and deceleration force trigger a complex neurometabolic response [48]. This response begins with an alteration of the neuronal cell membranes and axonal stretching, resulting in an abnormal flux of ions through ion channels and potential transient physical membrane defects [49]. This process will cause a significant release of neurotransmitters, especially excitatory amino acids (EAAs) [50], which may result in additional ionic flux. The Na1/K1 ATP-dependent pump is activated to reestablish ionic balance while depleting energy stores (**Figure 2**). This response may result in subsequent brain hypofunction and even permanent damage [52]. In brain concussion, these changes are generally considered self-limited and transient. However, some reports have shown that repeated brain injuries can have long-term consequences. The incapacity to deliver energy to the brain tissues after a concussion, combined with high energy requirements to restore damaged functions, results in an energy mismatch [47]. In response to the concussion cascade, pathophysiological events occur simultaneously, leading to potential changes in mental status, symptoms, cognitive function, or motor control.

In 2018, the first serum TBI marker test was approved by the US Food and Drug Administration [53]. The test was designed to detect the presence of two proteins in

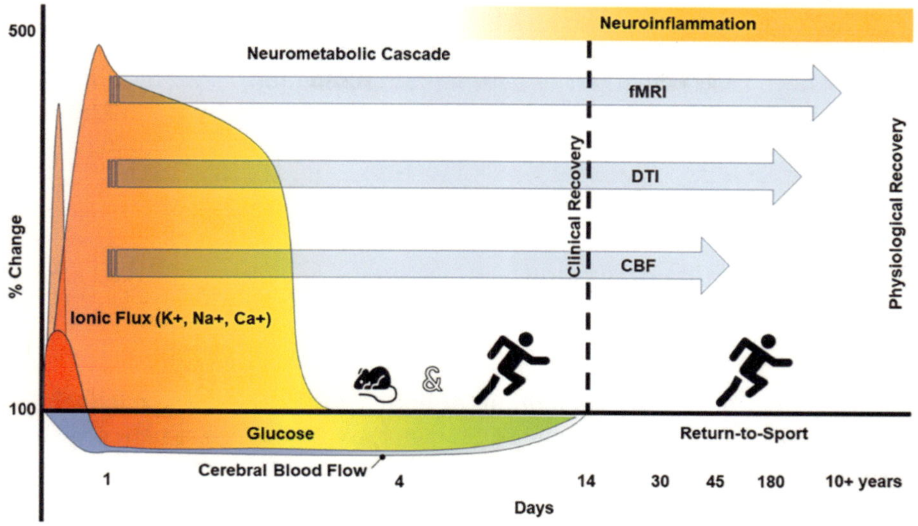

Figure 2.
Metabolic cascade indicates a gap between clinical recovery as defined as a return to pre-injury values on clinical measures of Sports-Related Concussion (SRC) in conjunction with a clinical examination and physiological recovery, which is defined as persisting physiological deficits despite achieving clinical recovery [51].

the brain: ubiquitin carboxy-terminal hydrolase-L1 (UCH-L1) and glial fibrillary acid protein (GFAP). However, other biomarkers are also under current investigation [52]. The calcium-binding protein S100B is a glial-specific protein found in the cytoplasm of astrocytes as the result of the breakdown of the BBB [54]. However, this biomarker has not been approved as a specific biomarker for TBI. Cytokine CCL11 is an inflammatory marker that is elevated in the cerebrospinal fluid (CSF) of individuals with chronic traumatic encephalopathy (CTE) [51, 55].

The neurofilament light polypeptide is an intermediate filament that can be found in the neuronal cytoskeleton and provides structural support to the axon. Interestingly, it has also been detected in the CSF of individuals who have suffered a TBI and may have a prognostic value [56]. Brain concussion patients often cannot remember the incident; therefore, these biomarkers may help physicians determine if a patient suffered this type of injury and may also quantify the severity of the injury. However, further research should be focused on the potential applications of these biomarkers.

Researchers hypothesize that pathophysiological changes that take place in the brain following a concussion are the result of neuronal depolarization, changes in glucose metabolism, excitatory neurotransmitter release, abnormal cerebral blood flow, and altered axonal function. These changes may occur concurrently at different stages after the injury [56].

In the pediatric age group, axonal myelination can affect the degree of disruption. Due to the ongoing myelination during the development of the brain, the axonal fibers and related microstructures could be more vulnerable to traumatic brain injuries in childhood compared with adults [57].

In animal models, inflammatory genes have been reported to upregulate acute neuroinflammatory responses [58]. Accordingly, a microglia and macrophage presence, as well as reactive astrogliosis, has been observed [59]. Therefore, inflammation could be a source of neuronal disruption following a brain concussion.

The larger concentrations of inflammatory markers in the brain could reduce behavioral responses and metabolites such as myo-inositol (mi.: an osmolyte). These have been used as markers of neuroinflammation [60]. Moreover, myo-isotol is an astrocyte activity marker that becomes hypertrophic during an inflammatory response to injury [61] and increases following concussion due to membrane damage [62].

6. Diagnosis of brain concussion

6.1 Clinical evaluation

The neurological signs and symptoms of brain concussion can be relatively subtle and transient. However, some patients may experience persistent sequelae, such as impaired attention and imbalance, which make them particularly vulnerable to new traumatisms. There is still no consensus on the definition of brain concussion or on its diagnostic criteria. In addition, there are no single specific assessments capable of identifying all patients with concussion, nor a minimum number of symptoms for its diagnosis [63, 64]. The diagnostic interview for brain concussion includes a history of the injury (sequence of the event and surrounding injury, intensity, memory), clinical evaluation (mental status after the impact), and risky factors (alcohol and drug use), which are useful tools in the diagnosis of brain concussion [65]. These are also useful in identifying patients at increased risk for severe or prolonged early impairments, neurologic catastrophe, or chronic neurobehavioral impairment [66]. Diagnostic tools can also be used to identify athletes with concussion-related early impairments and sports-related neurologic catastrophes (e.g., subdural hematoma).

Various standardized diagnostic tools may be used in the pre-hospital setting after an acute head injury to help determine the presence of a brain concussion. In athletes aged above 13 years, the Sideline Concussion Assessment Tool 5 (SCAT5) can be particularly useful. The memory assessment (Maddocks Questions) can be used in boys below the age of 12 years, whereas the Child-SCAT5 is a standardized tool for the evaluation of children between the ages of 5 and 12 years [47]. A recent report has shown that the Child SCAT5 was the most effective assessment tool for the differentiation between concussed and non-concussed middle school children.

It is also important to follow up with patients to detect any signs and symptoms of neurologic deterioration after the initial post-injury assessment, due to the frequent development of delayed symptoms and objective findings [67]. These signs and symptoms may include focal neurologic deficits, loss of consciousness, severe headaches, seizures, and altered mental status. If the patient deteriorates, it may indicate a more serious head injury and should be referred to an emergency department for further assessment [9].

6.2 Classification of brain concussion

At least 41 classification systems have been described to determine the severity and grade of a brain concussion. However, there is little consensus among professionals on the use of these systems in a clinical setting [68]. Many of these classifications rely on loss of consciousness and amnesia as their primary determinants for the severity of the traumatism:

- Cantu Scale [68]:
  - Grade I: Post-traumatic amnesia <30 min, no loss of consciousness.
  - Grade II: Loss of consciousness <5 min or amnesia lasting 30 min–24 h
  - Grade III: Loss of consciousness >5 min or amnesia >24 h
- Colorado Medical Society [69]:
  - Grade I: Confusion, no loss of consciousness
  - Grade II: Confusion, post-traumatic amnesia, no loss of consciousness.
  - Grade III: Loss of consciousness >5 min or amnesia >24 h.
- American Academy of Neurology guidelines [70, 71]:
  - Grade I: Confusion, symptoms last <15 min, no loss of consciousness
  - Grade II: Symptoms last >15 min, no loss of consciousness.
  - Grade III: Loss of consciousness (IIIa, coma lasts sec, IIIb for min)
- Other classifications of brain concussion also add medical imaging to their criteria (Available from: https://broadviewhealthcentre.com/concussion-grades-how-to-distinguish-degrees-of-concussions/):
  - Grade I (mild): Post-traumatic amnesia <24 h. Loss of consciousness 0–30 min, medical images normal, and symptoms: headache, dizziness, nausea.
  - Grade II (moderate): Post-traumatic amnesia >7 days. Loss of consciousness 30 min–24 h, medical images normal, and symptoms, headache, dizziness, and memory loss.
  - Grade III (severe): Post-traumatic amnesia 24 h–7 days. Loss of consciousness >24 h, medical images normal, and symptoms: headache, dizziness, memory loss, nausea, and difficulty focusing.

6.3 Neuroimaging and brain concussion

Brain concussion cannot be diagnosed with a routine computed tomogram (CT) scan or magnetic resonance imaging (MRI) scan. CT imaging should not be used to diagnose brain concussion. However, it can be performed to rule out more serious TBI, especially if there has been an associated LOC, post-traumatic amnesia, persistently altered mental status, focal neurologic deficit, evidence of a skull fracture on examination, or signs of clinical deterioration (Level C) [63]. Specific MRI sequences, such as diffusion tensor imaging and functional MRI, may result in an earlier diagnosis of concussion [72].

New advanced neuroimaging techniques may provide insights into the disrupted axonal structures. Diffusion Tensor Imaging (DTI) has been used to measure the diffusion properties of water, therefore providing a detailed view on how micro-structural tissues may function [73]. However, the use of advanced neuroimaging approaches for clinical purposes is not widely used. However, recent research is highlighting their potential use in the future [74, 75].

7. Treatment of brain concussion

The treatment for brain concussion typically includes bed rest and clinical monitoring for worsening of symptoms.

The use of helmets in brain concussion has shown no clear benefit in American football. Although athletes should be immediately removed from the game after a brain concussion, there is no evidence supporting absolute rest after a concussion [76]. Before the return to sports, athletes must initiate a progressive exercise program, be completely asymptomatic, and complete a standardized neuropsychological test. Moreover, a continuous evaluation for any recurring signs or symptoms should be performed. The recovery of pediatric and adolescent athletes is generally longer compared with older individuals [76]. Overall, the symptoms resolve in approximately 1–4 weeks. Finally, active rehabilitation may accelerate the recovery from a brain concussion.

8. Complications of brain concussion

Brain concussion may lead to serious long-term neurological effects, including impairments of cognitive functions, coordination, and social behavior [77].

8.1 Post-concussion syndrome

Post-concussion syndrome (PCS) is a heterogeneous condition that includes signs and symptoms of somatic, cognitive, and emotional domains. Whereas symptoms of concussion resolve in most individuals over days to weeks, in a small number of patients, symptoms could persist for months or years.

As mentioned earlier, the clinical consequences of concussion may present in an early post-traumatic stage as headache, dizziness, imbalance, fatigue, insomnia, impaired cognitive function, and phonophobia. However, late post-concussion symptoms may manifest as persistent somatic, emotional, and cognitive symptoms. This phase is highly affected by psychosocial factors. A successful treatment requires a thoughtful differential diagnosis that takes into account comorbidities and possible contributing factors. Its treatment should include a sequential approach that manages treatable symptoms that impact the functionality of the patient, such as depression, anxiety, insomnia, headache, musculoskeletal pain, and vertigo. In addition, the prescription of physical exercise is useful for disorders after a concussion [78].

9. Outcome

The outcome of a brain concussion is usually favorable [79]. The symptoms usually improve within the first one to two weeks. And the recovery timeframe after a concussion is typically 10 days [63]. The severity of the symptoms within the first few days after a head injury is the most consistent prognostic indicator [9]. However, there are still no definitive predictors for the recovery time after a concussion, and the anticipated recovery timeframe should be individualized for each patient [80].

Brain concussions are a public health problem that affect vulnerable populations, including young athletes, children, and the elderly. As awareness increases, more patients with acute concussions seek medical evaluations. The management of brain concussion includes a rapid removal from play, symptomatic treatment, and return to the sport with recommendations once the patient is asymptomatic. The inappropriate management of brain concussions may lead to recurrent injuries, prolonged recovery, and potential long-term sequelae. Understanding the key diagnostic features, post-injury assessment tools, symptomatic treatment, and management steps is essential for primary care providers [80, 81].

10. Future and research challenges

A universally agreed definition of brain concussion should be reached by professionals. Moreover, more robust diagnostic criteria based on neuroimaging or neurophysiological tests should be established. The diagnosis of post-concussion syndrome should be based on more objective criteria. These challenges should be addressed by a multidisciplinary international research team of expertise in brain concussion.

11. Conclusion

Concussion is the most common type of traumatic brain injury. However, there are different definitions and classification systems used to define this condition. The diagnosis is still based mainly on the clinical history and symptoms, which are often subjective. Neuroimaging and brain markers are not conclusive nor pathognomy of brain concussion. The diagnosis of post-concussion syndrome is based fundamentally on subjective symptoms, without objective standard parameters or neurophysiological or neuroimaging studies. Further investigations are needed for a better understanding of the brain concussion.

Author details

Ahmad Tamimi[1*], Iskandar Tamimi[2], Mohamad Barbarawi[3], Abdel Karim Qudah[4] and Faleh Tamimi[5]

1 Department of Neurosurgery, Faculty of Medicine, Jordan University Hospital, University of Jordan and Specialist Hospital, Amman, Jordan

2 Department of Orthopedic Surgery and Faculty of Medicine, University of Malaga, Spain

3 Department of Neurosurgery, Faculty of Medicine, Jordan University of Science and Technology, Irbid, Jordan

4 Pediatric Neurology, Faculty of Medicine, Jordan University Hospital University of Jordan and Jordan Hospital, Amman, Jordan

5 Faculty of Dentistry, Qatar University, Doha, Qatar

*Address all correspondence to: aftamimi@hotmail.com

References

[1] Masferrer R, Masferrer M, Prendergast V, Harrington TR. Grading scale for cerebral concussions. BNI Quarterly. Barrow Neurological Institute. 2000;**16**(1). ISSN 0894-5799

[2] McCrory PR, Ariens T, Berkovic SF. The nature and duration of acute concussive symptoms in Australian football. Clinical Journal of Sport Medicine. 2000;**10**(4):235-238

[3] Sivák Š et al. Early and delayed auditory oddball ERPs and brain MRI in patients with MTBI. Brain Injury. 2008;**22**(2):193-197

[4] McCrory PR, Berkovic SF. Concussion: The history of clinical and pathophysiological concepts and misconceptions. Neurology. 2001;**57**(12):2283-2289. DOI: 10.1212/wnl.57.12.2283

[5] Denny-Brown DE, Russell WR. Experimental concussion: (section of neurology). Proceedings of the Royal Society of Medicine. 1941;**34**(11):691-692

[6] Carroll L, Cassidy JD, Peloso P, Borg J, Von Holst H, Holm L, et al. Prognosis for mild traumatic brain injury: Results of the WHO collaborating Centre task force on mild traumatic brain injury. Journal of Rehabilitation Medicine. 2004;**36**(0):84-105

[7] Maas AIR et al. Standardizing data collection in traumatic brain injury. Journal of Neurotrauma. 2011;**28**(2):177-187

[8] Levin HS, Diaz-Arrastia RR. Diagnosis, prognosis, and clinical management of mild traumatic brain injury. The Lancet Neurology. 2015;**14**(5):506-517

[9] McCrory P et al. What is the definition of sports-related concussion: A systematic review. British Journal of Sports Medicine. 2017;**51**(11):877-887

[10] Agarwal N, Thakkar R, Than K. A concussion can affect memory, judgment, reflexes, speech, balance and muscle coordination. American Association of Neurological Surgeons; 29 April 2024. Available from: https://www.aans.org/en/Patients/Neurosurgical-Conditions-and-Treatments/Concussion

[11] Traumatic Brain Injury & Concussion. U.S Center for Disease Control and Prevention; 16 May 2024. Available from: https://www.cdc.gov/traumaticbraininjury/index.html

[12] Halstead ME et al. Sport-related concussion in children and adolescents. Pediatrics. 2018;**142**:6

[13] Whiteneck GG, Cuthbert JP, Corrigan JD, Bogner JA. Prevalence of self-reported lifetime history of traumatic brain injury and associated disability: A Statewide population-based survey. The Journal of Head Trauma Rehabilitation. 2016;**31**(1):E55-E62. DOI: 10.1097/HTR.0000000000000140

[14] Faul M, Xu L, Wald MM, et al. Traumatic Brain Injury in the United States: National Estimates of Prevalence and Incidence, 2002-2006 Injury Prevention 2010;16: A268

[15] Faul M, Coronado V. Epidemiology of traumatic brain injury. Handbook of Clinical Neurology. 2015;**127**:3-13

[16] Tagliaferri F, Compagnone C, Korsic M, Servadei F, Kraus JJAN. A systematic review of brain injury

epidemiology in Europe. Acta Neurochirurgica. 2006;**148**:255-268

[17] Kay A, Teasdale G. Head injury in the United Kingdom. World Journal of Surgery. 2001;**25**:1210-1220

[18] Lefevre-Dognin C, Cogné M, Perdrieau V, Granger A, Heslot C, Azouvi P. Definition and epidemiology of mild traumatic brain injury. Neurochirurgie. 2021;**67**(3):218-221

[19] Kelly JP, Nichols JS, Filley CM, Lillehei KO, Rubinstein D, Kleinschmidt-DeMasters BK. Concussion in sports. Guidelines for the prevention of catastrophic outcome. Journal of the American Medical Association. 1991;**266**(20):2867-2869. DOI: 10.1001/jama.266.20.2867

[20] Meehan WP, Taylor AM, Proctor M. The pediatric athlete: Younger athletes with sport-related concussion. Clinics in Sports Medicine. 2011;**30**(1):133-144

[21] Laker SR. Epidemiology of concussion and mild traumatic brain injury. PM&R. 2011;**3**:S354-S358

[22] Gordon KE, Dooley JM, Wood EP. Descriptive epidemiology of concussion. Pediatric Neurology. 2006;**34**(5):376-378. DOI: 10.1016/j.pediatrneurol.2005.09.007

[23] McCrory P, Meeuwisse W, Dvorak J, et al. Consensus statement on concussion in sport—The 5th international conference on concussion in sport held in Berlin, October 2016. British Journal of Sports Medicine. 2017;**51**:838-847

[24] Ropper AH, Gorson KC. Concussion. New England Journal of Medicine. 2007;**356**(2):166-172

[25] What Causes Traumatic Brain Injury. Eunice Kennedy Shriver National Institute of Child Health and Human Development. 2020. Available from: https://www.nichd.nih.gov/health/topics/tbi/conditioninfo/causes

[26] Concussion. Cleveland Clinic. 2024. Available from: https://my.clevelandclinic.org/health/diseases/15038-concussion

[27] Kakos BS, Young CC. Concussion Treatment & Management. Medscape. 05 Jun 2024. Available from: https://emedicine.medscape.com/article/92095-treatment

[28] Casson IR, Viano DC, Powell JW, Pellman EJ. Repeat concussions in the National Football League. Sports Health. 2011;**3**(1):11-24. DOI: 10.1177/1941738110391413

[29] Barry D. Jordan chronic traumatic brain injury associated with boxing. Seminars in Neurology. 2000;**20**(2):179-186. DOI: 10.1055/s-2000-9826

[30] Gerberich SG, Priest JD, Boen JR, Straub CP, Maxwell RE. Concussion incidences and severity in secondary school varsity football players. American Journal of Public Health. 1983;**73**(12):1370-1375

[31] Powell JW, Barber-Foss KD. Traumatic brain injury in high school athletes. JAMA. 1999;**282**(10):958-963

[32] Lowrance WW: Op. Cit. pp. 119-126. Negotiate Flexibly, but Explain Publicly, Nature No. 5540, January 22, 1976, p. 165

[33] Haddon W Jr. A logical framework for categorizing highway safety phenomena and activity. Journal of Trauma and Acute Care Surgery. 1972;**12**(3):193-207

[34] McKee AC, Robinson ME. Military-related traumatic brain injury and

neurodegeneration. Alzheimer's and Dementia. 2014;**10**:S242-S253

[35] Hoge CW, McGurk D, Thomas JL, Cox AL, Engel CC, Castro CA. Mild traumatic brain injury in US soldiers returning from Iraq. New England Journal of Medicine. 2008;**358**(5):453-463

[36] Young L, Rule GT, Bocchieri RT, Walilko TJ, Burns JM, Ling G. When physics meets biology: Low and high-velocity penetration, blunt impact, and blast injuries to the brain. Frontiers in Neurology. 2015;**6**:89. DOI: 10.3389/fneur.2015.00089

[37] Walker KR, Tesco G. Molecular mechanisms of cognitive dysfunction following traumatic brain injury. Frontiers in Aging Neuroscience. 2013;**5**:29

[38] Goldstein LE, Fisher AM, Tagge CA, Zhang XL, Velisek L, Sullivan JA, et al. Chronic traumatic encephalopathy in blast-exposed military veterans and a blast neurotrauma mouse model. Science Translational Medicine. 2012;**4**(134):134ra60-134ra60

[39] Bell RS, Vo AH, Neal CJ, Tigno J, Roberts R, Mossop C, et al. Military traumatic brain and spinal column injury: A 5-year study of the impact blast and other military-grade weaponry on the central nervous system. Journal of Trauma and Acute Care Surgery. 2009;**66**(4):S104-S111

[40] Duckworth JL, Grimes J, Ling GS. Pathophysiology of battlefield associated traumatic brain injury. Pathophysiology. 2013;**20**(1):23-30

[41] Roozenbeek B, Maas AI, Menon DK. Changing patterns in the epidemiology of traumatic brain injury. Nature Reviews Neurology. 2013;**9**(4):231-236

[42] Graham R, Rivara FP, Ford MA. Committee on Sports-Related Concussions in Youth; Board on Children, Youth, and Families; Institute of Medicine; Sports-Related Concussions in Youth: Improving the Science, Changing the Culture. Washington (DC): National Academies Press (US); 2014

[43] Paiva WS, Soares MS, Amorim RL, de Andrade AF, Matushita H, Teixeira MJ. Traumatic brain injury and shaken baby syndrome. Acta Médica Portuguesa. 2011;**24**(5):805-808

[44] Joyce T, Gossman W, Huecker MR. Pediatric abusive head trauma. In: StatPearls [Internet]. Treasure Island (FL): StatPearls Publishing; 2024. Available from: https://www.ncbi.nlm.nih.gov/books/NBK499836/ [Accessed: May 22, 2023]

[45] Harding B, Risdon RA, Krous HF. Shaken baby syndrome. BMJ. 2004;**328**(7442):720-721. DOI: 10.1136/bmj.328.7442.720

[46] Geddes JF, Vowles GH, Hackshaw AK, Nickols CD, Scott IS, Whitwell HL. Neuropathology of inflicted head injury in children: II microscopic brain injury in infants. Brain. 2001;**124**(7):1299-1306. DOI: 10.1093/brain/124.7.1299

[47] Howell DR, Wingerson MJ, Kirkwood MW, Grubenhoff JA, Wilson JC. Early aerobic exercise among adolescents at moderate/high risk for persistent post-concussion symptoms: A pilot randomized clinical trial. Physical Therapy in Sport. 2022;**55**:196-204

[48] Barkhoudarian G, Hovda DA, Giza CC. The molecular pathophysiology of concussive brain injury–an update. Physical Medicine and Rehabilitation Clinics. 2016;**27**(2):373-393

[49] Farkas O, Lifshitz J, Povlishock JT. Mechanoporation induced by diffuse traumatic brain injury: An irreversible or reversible response to injury? Journal of Neuroscience. 2006;**26**(12):3130-3140

[50] Katayama Y, Becker DP, Tamura T, Hovda DA. Massive increases in extracellular potassium and the indiscriminate release of glutamate following concussive brain injury. Journal of Neurosurgery. 1990;**73**(6):889-900

[51] Neumann KD, Broshek DK, Newman BT, Druzgal TJ, Kundu BK, Resch JE. Concussion: Beyond the cascade. Cells. 2023;**12**(17):2128

[52] Yoshino A, Hovda DA, Kawamata T, Katayama Y, Becker DP. Dynamic changes in local cerebral glucose utilization following cerebral concussion in rats: Evidence of a hyper-and subsequent hypometabolic state. Brain Research. 1991;**561**(1):106-119

[53] US Food and Drug Administration. 2018. Available from: https://www.fda.gov/NewsEvents/Newsroom/PressAnnouncements/ucm596531.htm. [Accessed: August 4, 2020]

[54] Berry JA, Elia C, Sweiss R, Lawandy S, Bowen I, Zampella B, et al. Pathophysiologic mechanisms of concussion, development of chronic traumatic encephalopathy, and emerging diagnostics: A narrative review. Journal of Osteopathic Medicine. 2020;**120**(9):582-589

[55] Al Nimer F, Thelin E, Nyström H, Dring AM, Svenningsson A, Piehl F, et al. Comparative assessment of the prognostic value of biomarkers in traumatic brain injury reveals an independent role for serum levels of neurofilament light. PLoS One. 2015;**10**(7):e0132177

[56] Giza C, Greco T, Prins ML. Concussion: Pathophysiology and clinical translation. Handbook of Clinical Neurology. 2018;**158**:51-61. DOI: 10.1016/b978-0-444-63954-7.00006-9

[57] Choe MC, Giza CC. Diagnosis and management of acute concussion. In: Seminars in Neurology. New York, NY, USA: Thieme Medical Publishers; 2015;**35**(1):029-041

[58] Li H, Zhang C, Yang C, Blevins M, Norris D, Zhao R, et al. C-terminal binding proteins 1 and 2 in traumatic brain injury-induced inflammation and their inhibition as an approach for anti-inflammatory treatment. International Journal of Biological Sciences. 2020;**16**(7):1107-1120. DOI: 10.7150/ijbs.42109

[59] Shultz SR, Bao F, Omana V, Chiu C, Brown A, Cain DP. Repeated mild lateral fluid percussion brain injury in the rat causes cumulative long-term behavioral impairments, neuroinflammation, and cortical loss in an animal model of repeated concussion. Journal of Neurotrauma. 2012;**29**(2):281-294

[60] Chang LC, Raty SR, Ortiz J, Bailard NS, Mathew SJ. The emerging use of ketamine for anesthesia and sedation in traumatic brain injuries. CNS Neuroscience & Therapeutics. 2013;**19**(6):390-395. DOI: 10.1111/cns.12077

[61] Albrecht JS, McCunn M, Stein DM, Simoni-Wastila L, Smith GS. Sex differences in mortality following isolated traumatic brain injury among older adults. The Journal of Trauma and Acute Care Surgery. 2016;**81**(3):486

[62] Henry LC, Tremblay S, Boulanger Y, Ellemberg D, Lassonde M. Neurometabolic changes in the acute phase after sports concussions correlate with symptom severity. Journal of Neurotrauma. 2010;**27**(1):65-76

[63] Ferry B, Means G, Green C, Risoli T, Martinez C, Vomer RP II, et al. Early initiation of vestibular therapy following sports-related concussions: A retrospective cohort study. Cureus. 2023;**15**(5):e3976

[64] Sussman ES, Ho AL, Pendharkar AV, Ghajar J. Clinical evaluation of concussion: The evolving role of oculomotor assessments. Neurosurgical Focus. 2016;**40**(4):E7. DOI: 10.3171/2016.1.FOCUS15610

[65] Silverberg ND, Iaccarino MA, Panenka WJ, et al. Management of Concussion and Mild Traumatic Brain Injury: A synthesis of practice guidelines. Archives of Physical Medicine and Rehabilitation. 2020;**101**(2):382-393. DOI: 10.1016/j.apmr.2019.10.179

[66] Giza CC, Kutcher JS, Ashwal S, Barth J, Getchius TS, Gioia GA, et al. Summary of evidence-based guideline update: Evaluation and management of concussion in sports: Report of the guideline development Subcommittee of the American Academy of neurology. Neurology. 2013;**80**(24):2250-2257. DOI: 10.1212/WNL.0b013e31828d57dd

[67] Putukian M. Clinical evaluation of the concussed athlete: A view from the sideline. Journal of Athletic Training. 2017;**52**(3):236-244

[68] Cantu RC, Gennarelli TA. History of concussion and chronic traumatic encephalopathy. In: Budson A, McKee AC, Cantu RC, Stern RA, editors. Chronic Traumatic Encephalopathy. Philadelphia, PA: Elsevier; 2017. pp. 1-18

[69] Silver JM, Hales RE, Yudofsky SC. Traumatic brain injury. In: Bourgeois JA, Hales RE, Young JS, Yudofsky SC, editors. The American Psychiatric Publishing Board Review Guide for Psychiatry. Washington, USA: American Psychiatric Publishing, Inc.; 2009. pp. 663-667

[70] Physiopedia. 2025. Available from: https://www.physio-pedia.com/Classification_of_Traumatic_Brain_Injury

[71] Practice Parameter: The Management of Concussion in Sports (Summary Statement) (PDF). American Academy of Neurology. [Accessed: January 28, 2008]

[72] Georges AM, Das J. Traumatic brain injury. In: StatPearls [Internet]. Treasure Island (FL): StatPearls Publishing; 2024. Available from: https://www.ncbi.nlm.nih.gov/books/NBK459300/ [Accessed: January 2, 2023]

[73] Shenton ME, Price BH, Levin L, Edersheim JG. Mild traumatic brain injury: Is DTI ready for the courtroom? International Journal of Law and Psychiatry. 2018;**61**:50-63

[74] Koerte IK, Hufschmidt J, Muehlmann M, et al. Advanced Neuroimaging of Mild Traumatic Brain Injury. In: Laskowitz D, Grant G, editors. Translational Research in Traumatic Brain Injury. Boca Raton (FL): CRC Press/Taylor and Francis Group; 2016. Chapter 13. Available from: https://www.ncbi.nlm.nih.gov/books/NBK326714/

[75] Jurick SM, Twamley EW, Crocker LD, Hays CC, Orff HJ, Golshan S, et al. Post concussive symptom over-reporting in Iraq/Afghanistan veterans with mild traumatic brain injury. Journal of Rehabilitation Research and Development. 2016;**53**(5):5-53(5):571-584

[76] Traumatic Brain Injury. 2023. Available from: https://msktc.org/sites/default/files/2023-07/23-22005-TBI-Booklet-combined-English-071023.pdf

[77] Danna-Dos-Santos A, Mohapatra S, Santos M, Degani AM. Long-term effects of mild traumatic brain injuries to oculomotor tracking performances

and reaction times to simple environmental stimuli. Scientific Reports. 2018;**8**(1):4583. DOI: 10.1038/s41598-018-22825-5

[78] Dwyer B, Katz DI. Post concussion syndrome. Handbook of Clinical Neurology. 2018;**158**:163-178. DOI: 10.1016/B978-0-444-63954-7.00017-3

[79] Harmon KG, Drezner J, Gammons M, Guskiewicz K, Halstead M, Herring S, et al. American medical Society for Sports Medicine position statement: Concussion in sport. Clinical Journal of Sport Medicine. 2013;**23**(1):1-18

[80] Collins MW, Kontos AP, Okonkwo DO, Almquist J, Bailes J, Barisa M, et al. Statements of agreement from the targeted evaluation and active management (TEAM) approaches to treating concussion meeting held in Pittsburgh, 2015. Neurosurgery. 2016;**79**(6):912-929

[81] Jackson WT, Starling AJ. Concussion evaluation and management. The Medical Clinics of North America. 2019;**103**(2):251-261. DOI: 10.1016/j.mcna.2018.10.005

Section 2

Pathophysiology and Biomarkers of TBI

Chapter 5

Perspective Chapter: Challenges in the Diagnosis of Post-Concussion Syndrome – Epidemiology, Pathophysiology, Neuropathology, Neuroimaging Biomarkers, and Salivary Biomarkers

Ioannis Mavroudis, Foivos Petridis, Alin Ciobica, Fatima Zahra Kamal and Manuela Padurariu

Abstract

Post-Concussion Syndrome (PCS) represents a complex constellation of symptoms that persist following a concussion or mild traumatic brain injury (mTBI), with significant implications for patient care and outcomes. Despite its prevalence, diagnosing PCS presents considerable challenges due to the subjective nature of symptoms, the absence of specific diagnostic tests, and the overlap with other neurological and psychiatric conditions. This review explores the multifaceted diagnostic challenges associated with PCS, including the heterogeneity of symptom presentation, the limitations of current neuroimaging techniques, and the overlap of PCS symptoms with other disorders. We also discuss the potential of emerging biomarkers and advanced imaging modalities to enhance diagnostic accuracy and provide a more objective basis for PCS identification. Additionally, the review highlights the importance of a multidisciplinary approach in both diagnosing and managing of PCS, integrating clinical evaluation with innovative diagnostic tools to improve patient outcomes. Through a comprehensive analysis of current practices and future directions, this review aims to shed light on the complexities of PCS diagnosis and pave the way for improved strategies in the identification and treatment of this condition.

Keywords: concussion, post-concussion syndrome, mild cognitive impairment, salivary biomarkers, micro-RNAs, tau protein, GFAP

1. Introduction

The term concussion, also known as mild traumatic brain injury (mTBI), lacks a universally accepted definition, reflecting diverse interpretations within the medical community [1]. The 2012 Zurich Consensus Statement on Concussion in Sport differentiates concussion from mTBI, describing it as a complex pathophysiological process affecting the brain, characterized by symptoms indicating a functional disturbance rather than structural damage [2]. These symptoms often resolve on their own and are not detectable through imaging. The American Academy of Neurology's 2013 guidelines, however, do not distinguish between TBI and concussion, instead defining it as a syndrome caused by biomechanical forces altering brain function, leading to changes in memory, orientation, and possibly consciousness [3].

Globally, TBI is a significant public health issue, being the leading cause of death and disability from trauma, with an estimated 69 million people affected annually worldwide. In the United States, mild cases represent 75% of the approximately 1.5 million TBIs each year [4].

Post-concussion syndrome (PCS) occurs after mild brain injuries, with a prevalence of 29–90% among head injury patients. It is characterized by symptoms like irritability, headaches, and concentration issues, which develop soon after the injury and can last for weeks to months. Persistent PCS is identified if symptoms continue beyond six months [5–10]. Diagnosis of PCS is complicated by the absence of objective findings and symptom variability, with criteria including a history of TBI and at least three specific symptoms such as insomnia and dizziness [11–13]. The DSM-5 categorizes PCS under neurocognitive disorders due to TBI, emphasizing the need for evidence of TBI and associated symptoms or neurological signs. Recent studies suggest PCS might involve long-term neurodegenerative processes, highlighting the potential for extended impacts beyond immediate neurological symptoms.

2. Post-concussion syndrome epidemiology

The diagnosis of Post-Concussion Syndrome (PCS) relies on two primary clinical frameworks: the Diagnostic and Statistical Manual of Mental Disorders, Fourth Edition (DSM-IV), 10th Revision (ICD-10), and the International Classification of Diseases. Although these criteria are useful, their application to identical populations can result in disparate outcomes, leading to divergent incidence rates documented in literature [14]. Research findings indicate that anywhere from 30 to 80% of individuals with mild to moderate traumatic brain injury (TBI) may display symptoms aligning with PCS (**Table 1**) [14].

Literature reviews have explored the link between TBI severity and PCS occurrence in individuals with mild TBI. Still, findings regarding the correlation between injury severity and PCS risk have been inconsistent. Factors considered in these analyses include the Glasgow Coma Scale (GCS) score at presentation, duration of consciousness loss, post-traumatic amnesia, and evidence of trauma on CT scans or MRI [14–18]. However, at least one study has identified a history of recent or multiple concussions as a significant risk factor for developing prolonged post-concussion symptoms [19].

Recent cohort studies and analyses have identified women as being particularly vulnerable to persistent PCS symptoms [14, 16, 20, 21]. Women are more prone to reporting symptoms such as irritability, headaches, concentration difficulties and fatigue. Additionally, increasing age is linked to a heightened PCS risk. In pediatric populations, gender-based symptom reporting differences have been noted, with female minors more frequently reporting symptoms and male minors more commonly experiencing loss of consciousness at injury time and seeking emergency

Symptom	Description
Headaches	Frequent and persistent, varying in intensity.
Dizziness	Sense of spinning or loss of balance.
Fatigue	Persistent tiredness not alleviated by rest.
Irritability	Increased frustration or anger with little provocation.
Sleep Disturbances	Difficulty falling or staying asleep; altered sleep patterns.
Memory and Concentration Difficulties	Problems with short-term memory and focusing on tasks.
Sensitivity to Light and Noise	Discomfort or increased symptoms in response to bright lights or loud sounds.

Table 1.
Common symptoms of post-concussion syndrome.

medical care. It is also posited that minors may have a lower PCS risk due to greater neuroplasticity compared to adults. While these observations primarily emerge from sports-related TBI research, experts suggest these patterns are likely applicable across various TBI causes [2].

3. Pathophysiology

The underlying mechanisms of concussion encompass metabolic disturbances, physiological alterations, and microstructural damage within the brain. Some research suggests a psychogenic origin for these symptoms, but it is likely that both biological and psychogenic factors significantly contribute to the development of Post-Concussion Syndrome (PCS) [22]. Symptoms associated with PCS often stem from damage to the autonomic nervous system, specifically affecting the white matter tracts that connect cortical control centers to the vagal nerve control through the spinal cord. Consequently, disruptions occur in both the sympathetic and parasympathetic nervous systems, often manifesting in symptoms reminiscent of depression. Damage to the autonomic nervous system can also disrupt cerebral blood flow, blood pressure, and heart rate regulation, which may manifest as dizziness, headaches, orthostatic intolerance, concentration difficulties, and confusion. The reduction in cerebral blood flow shortly after an injury can explain many PCS symptoms. In contrast, an elevation in cerebral blood flow following an injury can result in symptoms such as headaches, alterations in vision, dizziness, and intolerance to physical exertion. Moreover, fluctuations in heart rate due to damage in the vagal nerve tract can induce irregular spikes in blood pressure and heart rate during physical exertion, exacerbating premature fatigue [23].

Regarding the neurobiological aspects of PCS, both structural and biochemical alterations, including brain atrophy and regional volume loss, have been observed in animals and humans [24].

Psychogenic factors also play a role in PCS, as evidenced by empirical and clinical studies. The primary symptoms of PCS, such as headache, dizziness, and sleep disturbances, closely resemble the somatic manifestations seen in psychiatric disorders such as anxiety, depression, and post-traumatic stress disorder (PTSD). Moreover, the cognitive impairments associated with anxiety and depression closely resemble those seen in PCS, and these symptoms often improve following antidepressant therapy [25, 26].

4. Neuropathology of concussion

4.1 Diffuse axonal injury

Diffuse axonal injury (DAI) is a major neuropathological condition stemming from traumatic brain injury (TBI) due to shearing forces damaging the brain's axons [27–30]. It is mostly linked to moderate to severe TBI but also occurs in mild cases, with severity reflecting the force of impact (**Table 2**) [31, 32]. Traditional imaging techniques struggle to detect DAI, whereas advanced MRI, particularly diffusion tensor imaging (DTI), effectively identifies axonal damage, making it invaluable for diagnosing athletes with mild TBI from sports injuries [33–35]. Initially, DAI manifests as axonal shearing, leading to disrupted axonal transport, swelling, and ultimately, Wallerian degeneration [27].

Key in the progression of DAI is the disruption of axonal membranes, precipitating calcium influx, neurofilament compaction, and microtubule disassembly—processes primarily driven by calcium dysregulation and calpain activation, which breaks down essential cytoskeletal elements [36–39]. Blast injuries, significant in civilian and military contexts, lead to both immediate and long-term cognitive and psychiatric effects, with autopsy findings in veterans showing signs of chronic traumatic encephalopathy (CTE) similar to those in athletes with repeated concussions [40]. Symptoms include cognitive decline and emotional disturbances.

4.2 Microtubule disorganization

The disorganization of microtubules, stemming directly from the dynamic stretching of axons, leads to the immediate breakage and buckling of microtubules following injury [41]. This exacerbates the process of microtubule disassembly [41]. This disassembly leads to the accumulation of organelles within axons and subsequent swelling, ultimately resulting in axotomy and disconnection [36, 37]. Neuronal damage, characterized by swellings and axonal bulbs, is commonly found at the gray and

Neuropathological feature	Description
Diffuse Axonal Injury (DAI)	Shearing of brain axons due to acceleration/deceleration forces, leading to disrupted axonal transport and secondary degeneration.
Microtubule Disorganization	Immediate breakage and disassembly post-injury, causing axonal swelling and disconnection.
Role of Microglia	Activated microglia migrate to injured areas, potentially acting as a barrier and mediating inflammation.
Dendritic and Axonal Changes	Increased dendritic arborization and synaptogenesis indicating regenerative responses post-injury.
TDP-43 Protein Accumulation	Suggests involvement in mild TBI and CTE pathogenesis, representing a response to axonal damage.
Tau Protein Alterations	Critical in maintaining axonal cytoskeleton structure; changes correlate with neurodegeneration following TBI.

Table 2.
Neuropathology of post-concussion syndrome.

white matter interface within cortical sulci [42]. DTI studies link the DAI extent after mild TBI to cognitive issues post-concussion [43].

4.3 The role of microglia

Microglia are pivotal in the brain's immune response, mediating inflammation post-TBI. Research using animal models has demonstrated that activated microglia rapidly migrate towards areas of tissue damage, potentially serving as a protective barrier between unaffected and injured regions, highlighting their role in responding to axonal damage [44, 45]. This microglial activation involves the upregulation of inflammatory genes, chemokines, and mediators [46], though the therapeutic implications of modulating this response remain under exploration.

4.4 Dendritic and axonal changes

Post-TBI, dendritic and synaptic changes occur, including heightened synaptogenesis and dendritic branching, indicating a regenerative reaction [47]. Factors such as c-Jun and ATF-3 are linked to axonal regeneration post-DAI, with structural proteins like GAP-43 associated with neurite outgrowth from damaged axons after acute TBI phases [48, 49].

4.5 TDP-43 protein

The TAR DNA-binding protein 43 (TDP-43) accumulation, noted in athletes and boxers diagnosed with CTE following repeated brain trauma, suggests its involvement in the pathogenesis of both mTBI and CTE. The TDP-43 buildup, a common feature in various neurodegenerative diseases, could potentially serve as a physiological response to axonal damage [50–52]. Animal studies have indicated an increase in TDP-43 expression following TBI [50–52].

4.6 Tau protein

Tau protein is critical in maintaining axonal cytoskeleton structure within the central and peripheral nervous systems [53, 54]. While tau's primary presence is in the brain, it is also found in other tissues [55]. Research on TBI biomarkers has focused on tau variations, with studies showing tau level increases in cerebrospinal fluid and plasma following TBI, correlating with long-term outcomes [56–58]. Elevated tau levels have been documented in athletes and military personnel following concussions and blast exposures, respectively, with a connection between tau levels and neurological outcomes [59–76].

4.7 Inflammatory response

The inflammatory response in mild TBI involves activating immune cells and releasing pro- and anti-inflammatory mediators, with studies indicating early activation post-TBI that may persist for weeks or months. Biomarkers like IL-1, TNF-α, IL-6, and CRP have been linked to the severity and outcomes of mild TBI, highlighting inflammation's role in concussion pathophysiology and symptom persistence [77–84].

5. Neuroimaging biomarkers

5.1 Conventional MRI and DWI

In the study of Post-Concussion Syndrome (PCS), MRI and Diffusion-Weighted Imaging (DWI) reveal key differences in detecting brain abnormalities (**Tables 3** and **4**). Structural MRI is valuable for assessing brain damage, with T1-weighted sequences showing brain volume changes indicative of moderate to severe injuries. Notably, the anterior cingulate and left cingulate gyrus isthmus show atrophy, linked to cognitive deficits like impaired working memory [24], while the fusiform gyrus and ventromedial prefrontal cortex (vmPFC) volume correlate with emotional dysfunction in PCS, due to the vmPFC's connection to the amygdala [85, 86]. DWI is crucial for analyzing white matter integrity, focusing on mean diffusivity, axial diffusivity, radial diffusivity, and fractional anisotropy. Alterations in these parameters, particularly decreased fractional anisotropy and increased diffusivity, signify axonal injury in key tracts such as the corpus callosum, internal capsule, and longitudinal fasciculi [87–91]. These injuries affect cognitive functions, stemming from concussion-induced rotational forces [92]. Tractography enhances DWI by mapping structural connectivity, showing distinct patterns in PCS, especially between the hippocampus and striatum [93]. Structural neuroimaging has pinpointed the cingulate gyrus and prefrontal regions, alongside the corpus callosum and internal capsule, as critical areas affected in PCS. This variability reflects the diverse symptoms and populations studied, underscoring PCS's complexity [94].

5.2 Functional MRI

In functional MRI (fMRI) research, analyses either focus on Blood Oxygen Level Dependent (BOLD) activation levels or investigate the functional connectivity and network topology within the brain. These approaches offer insights into both normative and pathological brain states, with graph analysis metrics providing a sophisticated framework for understanding brain network topology in depth. This summary categorizes findings from Post-Concussion Syndrome (PCS) related fMRI studies under these analytical frameworks.

Biomarker	Type	Relevance
S100B	Serum	Indicates astroglial injury; elevated post-TBI.
GFAP	Serum/ CSF	Reflects astrocytic response to neuronal damage.
Tau Protein	Serum/ CSF	Associated with axonal injury; levels correlate with TBI severity.
Neurofilament Light Chain (NfL)	Serum/ CSF	Structural component indicating axonal injury and degeneration.
IL-1, IL-6, TNF-α	Serum	Inflammatory markers linked to severity and outcomes of TBI.

Table 3.
Serum and CSF biomarkers for post-concussion syndrome.

Biomarker Type	Description	Relevance to PCS
Conventional MRI and DWI	Detects structural changes in the brain.	Identifies anatomical and structural damage but may not capture subtle changes associated with PCS.
Diffusion Tensor Imaging (DTI)	Measures the diffusion of water molecules in brain tissue.	Highlights microstructural alterations in white matter tracts; sensitive to axonal injury.
Functional MRI (fMRI)	Assesses brain activity by detecting changes associated with blood flow.	Evaluates functional connectivity and neural activity patterns; useful for understanding cognitive impairments in PCS.
Magnetic Resonance Spectroscopy (MRS)	Non-invasive method to measure biochemical changes in the brain.	Provides insights into metabolic disturbances post-TBI; can detect neuronal injury and neuroinflammation.
Susceptibility Weighted Imaging (SWI)	Sensitive to magnetic susceptibility differences in tissue.	Detects microhemorrhages and iron deposits indicative of traumatic vascular injury.
Positron Emission Tomography (PET)	Imaging test that uses a radioactive substance to look for disease in the body.	Can identify metabolic abnormalities and neuroinflammation; potential for detecting tau pathology in CTE.

Table 4.
Neuroimaging biomarkers for post-concussion syndrome.

6. BOLD activation level analysis

Research has primarily examined deficits in selective attention and working memory, crucial cognitive domains affected after mild Traumatic Brain Injury (mTBI). Key brain regions implicated include the premotor area, dorsolateral and ventrolateral prefrontal cortex, posterior parietal area, supplementary motor area, and anterior cingulate cortex, with activation levels correlating with PCS severity [95–97]. Increased activation in the posterior cingulate cortex and the parahippocampal gyrus, associated with episodic memory, suggests a compensatory response to microstructural damage in PCS [96]. Additionally, the left angular gyrus shows hyperactivity to maintain working memory performance, indicating that PCS patients may utilize additional cognitive resources for task execution [98]. A noted decrease in activation within the medial prefrontal cortex, vital for emotion regulation and executive functions, suggests significant cognitive and affective impairments in PCS. Enhancements in this region's activity, possibly through transcranial magnetic stimulation, have been linked to reduced PCS symptoms [99–101]. Studies also highlight increased BOLD activity in response to visual stimuli in regions processing motion and objects, linking this to heightened sensitivity in PCS patients [102].

7. Functional connectivity analysis

Alterations in functional connectivity are evident across various networks in PCS, with reports of both hyperconnectivity and reduced whole-brain connectivity, particularly during the acute phase [103–105]. The Default Mode Network (DMN) and the thalamus are notably affected, with the DMN showing altered connectivity patterns that disrupt the balance between internal and external attention processes. Decreased connectivity in the DMN's posterior regions and altered interactions with the visual and left fronto-parietal networks are observed, alongside compensatory mechanisms in the medial prefrontal cortex to mitigate neurocognitive deficits [103, 106, 107]. Increased thalamo-cortical connectivity in PCS suggests inefficient neuronal activity, possibly due to changes in GABAergic inhibition, indicating disrupted modulatory interactions essential for cognitive and attentional functions [108–110].

8. Graph analysis

Graph analysis reveals topological changes in brain networks, highlighting alterations in modularity within temporal and frontal regions during different PCS phases. These changes, associated with executive functions and attention, are integrated with diffusion-weighted imaging to link functional network efficiency with diffuse axonal injury. Decreased local relative betweenness centrality in functional networks correlates with reduced fractional anisotropy, underscoring the impact of structural changes on network efficiency [109, 111–113].

9. Fluid biomarkers

9.1 Serum biomarkers

Fluid biomarkers offer a window into the pathophysiological processes activated by repeated head impacts, serving as vital tools for diagnosis, prognosis, and understanding the biological response to injury.

Among the serum biomarkers, neurofilament light polypeptide (NFL) is indicative of axonal injury in TBI. A study involving 19 American football athletes and an equal number of swim athletes highlighted the NFL increased levels in the football players, which notably did not normalize even nine months following the injury [113]. This persistence underscores the long-term impact of TBI on neural integrity.

Similarly, serum S-100 calcium-binding protein B and neuron-specific enolase (NSE) have been investigated for their roles in indicating astroglial and general neuronal injury, respectively, in PCS. In a study involving 47 preseason and 28 PCS professional ice hockey players, researchers noted an elevation in S100B levels among those with PCS, while NSE levels remained constant. This suggests that increases in S100B and NSE levels may also occur following physical exertion [106]. Another study, which compared 44 amateur boxers with 23 healthy controls, found elevated serum NSE levels in the boxers without concurrent changes in S100B levels [107], highlighting the differential response of these biomarkers to neurotrauma.

Further investigations into serum neurofilament H and SNTF have pointed towards their association with the neuronal axons stretch injury in TBI. In one study, SNTF and NFH heightened levels were detected in the sera of TBI patients undergoing surgical brain pressure release [72], while another study found elevated levels of SNTF in 28 concussed professional ice hockey players compared to 45 non-concussed players [114], suggesting their potential as diagnostic markers.

The significance of serum glial fibrillary acidic protein (GFAP) in reflecting the astrocytic response to neuronal damage was confirmed by a study involving 215 acute TBI patients, which observed elevated serum GFAP levels [115]. Additionally, serum interleukins (IL6, IL8) and tumor necrosis factor-alpha (TNF-α) have been linked to neuroinflammation in TBI. A study involving 24 TBI patients showed increased serum levels of these cytokines, possibly correlating with adverse outcomes and further brain damage [116].

9.2 Cerebrospinal fluid biomarkers

Turning to cerebrospinal fluid (CSF) biomarkers, research has illuminated the significance of YKL-40, GFAP, and amyloid β40, β42 in PCS, with a study reporting YKL-40 and GFAP increased levels, alongside Aβ40 and Aβ42 decreased in 28 PCS professional athletes compared to 19 controls [117]. This suggests a specific glial response to injury.

Following a similar pattern, heightened levels of NF light protein and diminished amyloid β CSF levels were detected in 16 ice hockey players diagnosed with PCS, in contrast to 15 control individuals [118], pointing towards axonal injury and the potential disturbance of amyloid processing.

Moreover, CSF total tau levels have been scrutinized for their correlation with axonal injury in TBI. Research with 68 former NFL players revealed that elevated CSF total tau levels correlated with the cumulative head impact index [119], suggesting a direct link between repeated head impacts and tau pathology. The study also found increased levels of sTREM2 in the CSF of these players, significantly associated with elevated CSF T-tau levels [119], pointing to microglial activation in response to repeated concussions.

Inflammatory markers in the CSF, such as IL1 and IL6, have been shown to correlate with TBI severity. In a study involving 37 severe TBI patients, elevated levels of these cytokines were observed, and they were associated with outcomes as assessed by the Glasgow Outcome Scale [120], highlighting the inflammatory cascade triggered by severe head injuries.

This body of research underscores the potential of fluid biomarkers in advancing our understanding of TBI and PCS. By quantifying specific proteins and cytokines, clinicians and researchers can gain insights into the molecular and cellular responses to brain injury, paving the way for improved diagnostic criteria, prognostic assessments, and the development of targeted therapies. As the field progresses, these biomarkers hold the promise of elucidating the complex landscape of neurotrauma, offering hope for more effective management and treatment strategies for those affected by TBI and its long-lasting consequences.

9.3 Salivary biomarkers

Although seemingly unrelated to the saliva's primary functions, salivary molecules can serve as potent indicators of local and systemic health issues despite their roles not being fully understood yet [121]. The utility of saliva in molecular diagnostics is particularly appealing due to its non-invasive, cost-effective collection, transportation, and processing advantages. The diagnostic potential of saliva has been highlighted, given its inclusion of serum constituents that migrate from the salivary glands' local vasculature into the gingival fluid flow, as discussed by Kaufman and Lamster [122]. This allows for the cost-effective assessment of systemic disease biomarkers by acquiring viable biological fluid samples with minimal effort, training, risk, and discomfort. Furthermore, saliva sampling is the preferred method for repeat collections among patients undergoing biological fluid sample collection [123]. It has been recognized as a viable source for complex molecular assessments like DNA sequencing compared to blood samples [124]. Lucía Melguizo-Rodríguez [125] identified over thirty-five salivary biomarkers specific to oral diseases, and transcriptomics studies have revealed more than 3000 mRNA species and over 300 miRNAs [126].

The challenge in diagnosing TBIs, particularly due to the brain tissue lesions caused by concussions, necessitates early identification of potential brain damage following mild head impacts [127]. Recent literature primarily focuses on blood and CSF biomarkers, such as S100B protein, GFAP, neurofilament light chain, α-II spectrin, UCHL-1, tau protein, and γ-enolase whose levels are altered after head traumas [128, 129]. Although not disease-specific, these biomarkers indicate the brain's response to injury and stress. The ongoing search for TBI, PCS, and CTE-specific biomarkers highlights the need for fast, reliable, and non-invasive diagnostic methods, with recent studies suggesting saliva as a promising medium for concussion and TBI diagnostics [125, 126].

In the context of TBI and PCS diagnostics, emerging research on salivary biomarkers underscores their diagnostic significance [130]. The discussion surrounding the extracranial origins of these biomarkers highlights blood-brain barrier permeability as a potential constraint for blood-based biomarkers. This limitation may not apply to salivary biomarkers. Understanding how central nervous system-produced molecules reach the saliva is crucial [130], with Murcko et al. [131] suggesting various distribution pathways beyond typical tissue damage or blood-brain barrier disruption. Saliva has been shown to contain microRNA, S100B, NfL, and extracellular vesicles associated with traumatic events [125, 126, 130], indicating its potential as a diagnostic tool for TBI and PCS.

S100 proteins, including S100B, play roles in various physiological processes and are found in the muscles, central nervous system, and vascular endothelium, with both intracellular and extracellular functions [130, 131]. S100B's interaction with RAGE receptors is crucial for its role in neuroinflammation [132], and its signaling pathways are involved in cellular responses to stress and gene expression [133]. Despite S100B being present in multiple organs, its clinical significance remains intact following a TBI-induced blood-brain barrier disruption [130]. Salivary S100B levels, significantly higher than blood levels irrespective of pathology [134] and effective in differentiating TBI patients from control subjects [135], highlight its potential as an alternative diagnostic biomarker for TBI. However, its association with head impact exposure remains to be conclusively demonstrated [136].

Neurofilament light chain (NfL), abundant in the nervous system, serves as a structural component and a biomarker for neurodegenerative conditions, reflecting axonal injury and degeneration [137, 138]. Its increased levels in peripheral fluids suggest significant nerve damage [139], with studies linking serum NfL levels to TBI severity and PCS extent [140]. Salivary NfL, potentially indicating axonal injury following repeated head impacts [136], emphasizes the diagnostic relevance of saliva in TBI and PCS.

MicroRNAs in saliva offer a non-invasive diagnostic avenue for mild TBI and PCS [141], with studies demonstrating their predictive value for TBI and association with post-concussion symptoms [142, 143]. The expression of salivary miRNAs, alongside neurocognitive testing, enhances the diagnostic accuracy for mild TBI [144], suggesting their utility in distinguishing between concussed and non-concussed individuals [145, 146].

Extracellular vesicles (EVs), as carriers of cellular communication, play roles in protein dissemination and pathological protein spread in conditions like TBI [147, 148]. Salivary EVs have been explored as biomarkers for mild TBI, revealing genetic overlaps with Alzheimer's disease and illustrating the potential of saliva in TBI diagnostics [149, 150].

This exploration into salivary biomarkers enriches our understanding of TBI diagnostics, indicating a promising future for non-invasive, saliva-based detection methods that could revolutionize diagnosing and understanding TBIs and their long-term impacts.

10. Post-concussion syndrome diagnostic challenges

The Post-Concussion Syndrome (PCS) diagnosis presents significant challenges to clinicians due to the heterogeneity of symptoms, the absence of definitive diagnostic tests, and the overlap with other conditions. These challenges complicate the clinical management and treatment of PCS, necessitating a nuanced approach to diagnosis.

10.1 Heterogeneity of symptoms

PCS symptoms are highly variable and subjective, including headaches, dizziness, fatigue, irritability, and cognitive disturbances. This variability poses a diagnostic challenge, as there is no single symptom or objective finding that definitively confirms PCS. The subjective nature of many symptoms further complicates diagnosis, as similar symptoms can be reported in other conditions, such as chronic pain syndromes, depression, and anxiety disorders.

10.2 Lack of definitive diagnostic tests

Currently, there are no definitive imaging or laboratory tests for PCS. Conventional neuroimaging techniques, such as CT and standard MRI, often fail to detect the subtle brain changes associated with PCS. Advanced imaging techniques like functional MRI (fMRI) and diffusion tensor imaging (DTI) show promise in identifying microstructural and functional brain changes, respectively, but are not routinely available in clinical practice. Moreover, these imaging findings are not specific to PCS and can be observed in other neurological conditions.

10.3 Overlap with other conditions

PCS shares symptoms with several other conditions, including migraine headaches, depression, anxiety disorders, and chronic pain syndromes. This overlap can lead to misdiagnosis or underestimation of the impact of concussive injury on the patient's symptoms. Differentiating PCS from these conditions is crucial for appropriate management but requires careful clinical evaluation and, often, a multidisciplinary approach.

10.4 Reliance on clinical criteria

The PCS diagnosis relies on clinical standards, such as those delineated in the ICD-10 and DSM-5. While these criteria provide a framework for diagnosis, their application can be subjective and depends on the clinician's judgment. The reliance on clinical criteria without objective biomarkers for PCS adds to the diagnostic uncertainty.

10.5 Emerging biomarkers

Research into fluid biomarkers, including serum and cerebrospinal fluid (CSF) biomarkers, offers hope for more objective diagnostic criteria in the future. Biomarkers such as S100B, GFAP, and tau protein have been associated with brain injury and PCS. However, these biomarkers are not yet widely available for clinical use and require further validation to determine their diagnostic utility in PCS.

11. Conclusion

The diagnostic challenges of PCS require clinicians to adopt a comprehensive, multidisciplinary approach that considers the broad spectrum of symptoms and the potential overlap with other conditions. Advances in imaging and biomarker research hold promise for improving the diagnostic process, but until these advances are integrated into clinical practice, the diagnosis of PCS will remain a clinical challenge based on a combination of patient history, symptomatology, and exclusion of other conditions.

Author details

Ioannis Mavroudis[1,2]*, Foivos Petridis[3], Alin Ciobica[4,5,6,7], Fatima Zahra Kamal[8] and Manuela Padurariu[9]

1 Department of Neuroscience, Leeds Teaching Hospitals, NHS Trust, Leeds, UK

2 Leeds University, Leeds, UK

3 Third Department of Neurology, Aristotle University of Thessaloniki, Greece

4 Department of Biology, Faculty of Biology, Alexandru Ioan Cuza University of Iasi, Iasi, Romania

5 Centre of Biomedical Research, Romanian Academy, Iasi, Romania

6 Academy of Romanian Scientists, Bucharest, Romania

7 Preclinical Department, Apollonia University, Iasi, Romania

8 Higher Institute of Nursing Professions and Health Technical (ISPITS), Marrakech, Morocco

9 "Socola" Institute of Psychiatry, Iași, Romania

*Address all correspondence to: ioannis.mavroudis@gmail.com

References

[1] Sharp DJ, Jenkins PO. Concussion is confusing us all. Practical Neurology. 2015;**15**(3):172-186. DOI: 10.1136/practneurol-2015-001087

[2] McCrory P, Meeuwisse WH, Aubry M, et al. Consensus statement on concussion in sport: The 4th international conference on concussion in sport held in Zurich, November 2012. British Journal of Sports Medicine. 2013;**47**:250-258. DOI: 10.1136/bjsports-2013-092313

[3] Giza CC, Kutcher JS, Ashwal S, et al. Summary of evidence-based guideline update: Evaluation and management of concussion in sports: Report of the guideline development Subcommittee of the American Academy of neurology. Neurology. 2013;**80**:2250-2257. DOI: 10.1212/WNL.0b013e31828d57dd

[4] Rubiano AM, Carney N, Chesnut R, Puyana JC. Global neurotrauma research challenges and opportunities. Nature. 2015;**527**:S193-S197. DOI: 10.1038/nature16035

[5] McKee AC, Cantu RC, Nowinski CJ, Hedley-Whyte ET, Gavett BE, Budson AE, et al. Chronic traumatic encephalopathy in athletes: Progressive tauopathy after repetitive head injury. Journal of Neuropathology and Experimental Neurology. 2009;**68**:709-735. DOI: 10.1097/NEN.0b013e3181a9d503

[6] McKee AC, Gavett BE, Stern RA, Nowinski CJ, Cantu RC, Kowall NW, et al. TDP-43 proteinopathy and motor neuron disease in chronic traumatic encephalopathy. Journal of Neuropathology and Experimental Neurology. 2010;**69**:918-929. DOI: 10.1097/NEN.0b013e3181ee7d85

[7] McKee AC, Stern RA, Nowinski CJ, Stein TD, Alvarez VE, Daneshvar DH, et al. The spectrum of disease in chronic traumatic encephalopathy. Brain. 2013;**136**:43-64. DOI: 10.1093/brain/aws307

[8] Hof PR, Knabe R, Bovier P, Bouras C. Neuropathological observations in a case of autism presenting with self-injury behavior. Acta Neuropathologica. 1991;**82**:321-326. DOI: 10.1007/BF00308819

[9] Geddes JF, Vowles GH, Nicoll JA, Revesz T. Neuronal cytoskeletal changes are an early consequence of repetitive head injury. Acta Neuropathologica. 1999;**98**:171-178. DOI: 10.1007/s004010051066

[10] Goldstein LE, Fisher AM, Tagge CA, Zhang XL, Velisek L, Sullivan JA, et al. Chronic traumatic encephalopathy in blast-exposed military veterans and a blast neurotrauma mouse model. Science Translational Medicine. 2012;**4**:134-160. DOI: 10.1126/scitranslmed.3003716

[11] Jellinger KA. Basic mechanisms of neurodegeneration: A critical update. Journal of Cellular and Molecular Medicine. 2010;**14**:457-487. DOI: 10.1111/j.1582-4934.2010.01010.x

[12] Ontario Neurotrauma Foundation Guideline for Concussion/Mild Traumatic Brain Injury & Prolonged Symptoms (3rd Edition), For Adults Over 18 Years of Age. Available from: https://braininjuryguidelines.org/concussion/ (accessed 19 January 2022)

[13] Reuben A, Sampson P, Harris AR, Williams H, Yates P. Postconcussion syndrome (PCS) in the emergency department: Predicting and pre-empting

persistent symptoms following a mild traumatic brain injury. Emergency Medicine Journal. 2014;**31**:72-77. DOI: 10.1136/emermed-2012-201667

[14] McCauley SR, Boake C, Pedroza C, Brown SA, Levin HS, Goodman HS, et al. Postconcussional disorder: Are the DSM-IV criteria an improvement over the ICD-10? The Journal of Nervous and Mental Disease. 2005;**193**(8):540-550

[15] Haas DC. Chronic post-traumatic headaches classified and compared with natural headaches. Cephalalgia. 1996;**16**(7):486-493

[16] de Kruijk JR, Leffers P, Meerhoff S, Rutten J, Twijnstra A. Effectiveness of bed rest after mild traumatic brain injury: A randomised trial of no versus six days of bed rest. Journal of Neurology, Neurosurgery, and Psychiatry. 2002;**73**(2):167-172

[17] Hughes DG, Jackson A, Mason DL, Berry E, Hollis S, Yates DW. Abnormalities on magnetic resonance imaging seen acutely following mild traumatic brain injury: Correlation with neuropsychological tests and delayed recovery. Neuroradiology. 2004;**46**(7):550-558

[18] McCauley SR, Boake C, Levin HS, Contant CF, Song JX. Postconcussional disorder following mild to moderate traumatic brain injury: Anxiety, depression, and social support as risk factors and comorbidities. Journal of Clinical and Experimental Neuropsychology. 2001;**23**(6):792-808

[19] Eisenberg MA, Andrea J, Meehan W, Mannix R. Time interval between concussions and symptom duration. Pediatrics. 2013;**132**(1):8-17

[20] Bazarian JJ, Atabaki S. Predicting postconcussion syndrome after minor traumatic brain injury. Academic Emergency Medicine. 2001;**8**(8):788-795

[21] Fenton G, McClelland R, Montgomery A, MacFlynn G, Rutherford W. The postconcussional syndrome: Social antecedents and psychological sequelae. The British Journal of Psychiatry. 1993;**162**:493-497

[22] Lishman WA. Physiogenesis and psychogenesis in the 'post-concussional syndrome'. The British Journal of Psychiatry. 1988 Oct;**153**:460-469

[23] Leddy J, Baker JG, Haider MN, Hinds A, Willer B. A physiological approach to prolonged recovery from sport-related concussion. Journal of Athletic Training. 2017;**52**(3):299-308

[24] Zhou Y, Kierans A, Kenul D, Ge Y, Rath J, Reaume J, et al. Mild traumatic brain injury: Longitudinal regional brain volume changes. Radiology. 2013;**267**(3):880-890

[25] Brand N, Jolles J. Information processing in depression and anxiety. Psychological Medicine. 1987;**17**(1):145-153

[26] Nicholson K, Martelli MF, Zasler ND. Does pain confound interpretation of neuropsychological test results? NeuroRehabilitation. 2001;**16**(4):225-230

[27] Johnson VE, Stewart W, Smith DH. Axonal pathology in traumatic brain injury. Experimental Neurology. 2013;**246**:35-43

[28] Meaney DF, Smith DH, Shreiber DI, et al. Biomechanical analysis of experimental diffuse axonal injury. Journal of Neurotrauma. 1995;**12**:689-694

[29] Adams JH, Doyle D, Ford I, Gennarelli TA, Graham DI,

McLellan DR. Diffuse axonal injury in head injury: Definition, diagnosis and grading. Histopathology. 1989;**15**(1):49-59. DOI: 10.1111/j.1365-2559.1989.tb03040.x

[30] Alexander MP. Mild traumatic brain injury: Pathophysiology, natural history, and clinical management. Neurology. 1995;**45**(7):1253-1260. DOI: 10.1212/wnl.45.7.1253

[31] Oppenheimer DR. Microscopic lesions in the brain following head injury. Journal of Neurology, Neurosurgery, and Psychiatry. 1968;**31**(4):299-306. DOI: 10.1136/jnnp.31.4.299

[32] Elson LM, Ward CC. Mechanisms and pathophysiology of mild head injury. Seminars in Neurology. 1994;**14**(1):8-18. DOI: 10.1055/s-2008-1041053

[33] Bazarian JJ, Zhong J, Blyth B, Zhu T, Kavcic V, Peterson D. Diffusion tensor imaging detects clinically important axonal damage after mild traumatic brain injury: A pilot study. Journal of Neurotrauma. 2007;**24**(9):1447-1459. DOI: 10.1089/neu.2007.0241

[34] Mayer AR, Ling J, Mannell MV, Gasparovic C, Phillips JP, Doezema D, et al. A prospective diffusion tensor imaging study in mild traumatic brain injury. Neurology. 2010;**74**(8):643-650. DOI: 10.1212/WNL.0b013e3181d0ccdd

[35] Bazarian JJ, Zhu T, Blyth B, Borrino A, Zhong J. Subject-specific changes in brain white matter on diffusion tensor imaging after sports-related concussion. Magnetic Resonance Imaging. 2012;**30**(2):171-180. DOI: 10.1016/j.mri.2011.10.001

[36] Giza CC, Hovda DA. The neurometabolic cascade of concussion. Journal of Athletic Training. 2001;**36**(3):228-235

[37] Barkhoudarian G, Hovda DA, Giza CC. The molecular pathophysiology of concussive brain injury. Clinics in Sports Medicine. 2011;**30**(1):33-48. DOI: 10.1016/j.csm.2010.09.001

[38] McCracken E, Hunter AJ, Patel S, Graham DI, Dewar D. Calpain activation and cytoskeletal protein breakdown in the corpus callosum of head-injured patients. Journal of Neurotrauma. 1999;**16**(9):749-761. DOI: 10.1089/neu.1999.16.749

[39] Saatman KE, Creed J, Raghupathi R. Calpain as a therapeutic target in traumatic brain injury. Neurotherapeutics. 2010;**7**(1):31-42. DOI: 10.1016/j.nurt.2009.11.002

[40] Mavroudis I, Kazis D, Chowdhury R, Petridis F, Costa V, Balmus IM, et al. Post-concussion syndrome and chronic traumatic encephalopathy: Narrative review on the neuropathology, neuroimaging and fluid biomarkers. Diagnostics (Basel). 2022;**12**(3):740. DOI: 10.3390/diagnostics12030740

[41] Tang-Schomer MD, Patel AR, Baas PW, Smith DH. Mechanical breaking of microtubules in axons during dynamic stretch injury underlies delayed elasticity, microtubule disassembly, and axon degeneration. The FASEB Journal. 2010;**24**(5):1401-1410. DOI: 10.1096/fj.09-142844

[42] Chen XH, Siman R, Iwata A, Meaney DF, Trojanowski JQ, Smith DH. Long-term accumulation of amyloid-beta, beta-secretase, presenilin-1, and caspase-3 in damaged axons following brain trauma. The American Journal of Pathology. 2004;**165**(2):357-371. DOI: 10.1016/s0002-9440(10)63303-2

[43] Lipton ML, Gellella E, Lo C, Gold T, Ardekani BA, Shifteh K, et al. Multifocal white matter ultrastructural

abnormalities in mild traumatic brain injury with cognitive disability: A voxel-wise analysis of diffusion tensor imaging. Journal of Neurotrauma. 2008;**25**(11):1335-1342. DOI: 10.1089/neu.2008.0547

[44] Davalos D, Grutzendler J, Yang G, Kim JV, Zuo Y, Jung S, et al. ATP mediates rapid microglial response to local brain injury in vivo. Nature Neuroscience. 2005;**8**(6):752-758. DOI: 10.1038/nn1472

[45] Shitaka Y, Tran HT, Bennett RE, Sanchez L, Levy MA, Dikranian K, et al. Repetitive closed-skull traumatic brain injury in mice causes persistent multifocal axonal injury and microglial reactivity. Journal of Neuropathology and Experimental Neurology. 2011;**70**(7):551-567. DOI: 10.1097/NEN.0b013e31821f891f

[46] Ziebell JM, Morganti-Kossmann MC. Involvement of pro- and anti-inflammatory cytokines and chemokines in the pathophysiology of traumatic brain injury. Neurotherapeutics. 2010;**7**(1):22-30. DOI: 10.1016/j.nurt.2009.10.016

[47] Keyvani K, Schallert T. Plasticity-associated molecular and structural events in the injured brain. Journal of Neuropathology and Experimental Neurology. 2002;**61**(10):831-840. DOI: 10.1093/jnen/61.10.831

[48] Greer JE, McGinn MJ, Povlishock JT. Diffuse traumatic axonal injury in the mouse induces atrophy, c-Jun activation, and axonal outgrowth in the axotomized neuronal population. The Journal of Neuroscience. 2011;**31**(13):5089-5105. DOI: 10.1523/JNEUROSCI.5103-10.2011

[49] Christman CW, Salvant JB Jr, Walker SA, Povlishock JT. Characterization of a prolonged regenerative attempt by diffusely injured axons following traumatic brain injury in adult cat: A light and electron microscopic immunocytochemical study. Acta Neuropathologica. 1997;**94**(4):329-337. DOI: 10.1007/s004010050715

[50] Neumann M, Sampathu DM, Kwong LK, Truax AC, Micsenyi MC, Chou TT, et al. Ubiquitinated TDP-43 in frontotemporal lobar degeneration and amyotrophic lateral sclerosis. Science. 2006;**314**(5796):130-133. DOI: 10.1126/science.1134108

[51] Kadokura A, Yamazaki T, Lemere CA, Takatama M, Okamoto K. Regional distribution of TDP-43 inclusions in Alzheimer disease (AD) brains: Their relation to AD common pathology. Neuropathology. 2009;**29**(5):566-573. DOI: 10.1111/j.1440-1789.2009.01017.x

[52] King A, Sweeney F, Bodi I, Troakes C, Maekawa S, Al-Sarraj S. Abnormal TDP-43 expression is identified in the neocortex in cases of dementia pugilistica, but is mainly confined to the limbic system when identified in high and moderate stages of Alzheimer's disease. Neuropathology. 2010;**30**(4):408-419. DOI: 10.1111/j.1440-1789.2009.01085.x

[53] Olivera A, Lejbman N, Jeromin A, et al. Peripheral Total tau in military personnel who sustain traumatic brain injuries during deployment. JAMA Neurology. 2015;**72**:1109

[54] Rubenstein R, Chang B, Davies P, Wagner AK, Robertson CS, Wang KKW. A novel, ultrasensitive assay for tau: Potential for assessing traumatic brain injury in tissues and biofluids. Journal of Neurotrauma. 2015;**32**:342-352

[55] Hanes J, Zilka N, Bartkova M, Caletkova M, Dobrota D, Novak M. Rat tau proteome consists of six tau isoforms:

Implication for animal models of human tauopathies. Journal of Neurochemistry. 2009;**108**:1167-1176

[56] Zetterberg H, Smith DH, Blennow K. Biomarkers of mild traumatic brain injury in cerebrospinal fluid and blood. Nature Reviews. Neurology. 2013;**9**:201-210

[57] Morris M, Maeda S, Vossel K, Mucke L. The many faces of tau. Neuron. 2011;**70**:410-426

[58] Shahim P, Gill JM, Blennow K, Zetterberg H. Fluid biomarkers for chronic traumatic encephalopathy. Seminars in Neurology. 2020;**40**:411-419

[59] Ost M, Nylén K, Csajbok L, et al. Initial CSF total tau correlates with 1-year outcome in patients with traumatic brain injury. Neurology. 2006;**67**:1600-1604

[60] Franz G, Beer R, Kampfl A, et al. Amyloid beta 1-42 and tau in cerebrospinal fluid after severe traumatic brain injury. Neurology. 2003;**60**:1457-1461

[61] Neselius S, Brisby H, Theodorsson A, Blennow K, Zetterberg H, Marcusson J. CSF-biomarkers in Olympic boxing: Diagnosis and effects of repetitive head trauma. PLoS One. 2012;7:e33606

[62] Zetterberg H, Hietala MA, Jonsson M, et al. Neurochemical aftermath of amateur boxing. Archives of Neurology. 2006;**63**:1277-1280

[63] Kawata K, Liu CY, Merkel SF, Ramirez SH, Tierney RT, Langford D. Blood biomarkers for brain injury: What are we measuring? Neuroscience and Biobehavioral Reviews. 2016;**68**:460-473

[64] Mattsson N, Zetterberg H, Janelidze S, et al. Plasma tau in Alzheimer disease. Neurology. 2016;**87**:1827-1835

[65] Ledreux A, Pryhoda MK, Gorgens K, et al. Assessment of long-term effects of sports-related concussions: Biological mechanisms and exosomal biomarkers. Frontiers in Neuroscience. 2020;**14**:761

[66] Hossain I, Mohammadian M, Takala RSK, et al. Admission levels of total tau and β-amyloid isoforms 1-40 and 1-42 in predicting the outcome of mild traumatic brain injury. Frontiers in Neurology. 2020;**11**:325

[67] Rubenstein R, Chang B, Yue JK, et al. Comparing plasma phospho tau, total tau, and phospho tau–total tau ratio as acute and chronic traumatic brain injury biomarkers. JAMA Neurology. 2017;**74**:1063

[68] Walker A, Chapin B, Abisambra J, DeKosky ST. Association between single moderate to severe traumatic brain injury and long-term tauopathy in humans and preclinical animal models: A systematic narrative review of the literature. Acta Neuropathologica Communications. 2022;**10**:1-20

[69] Blomberg M, Jensen M, Basun H, Lannfelt L, Wahlund LO. Cerebrospinal fluid tau levels increase with age in healthy individuals. Dementia and Geriatric Cognitive Disorders. 2001;**12**:127-132

[70] Mondello S, Guedes VA, Lai C, Jeromin A, Bazarian JJ, Gill JM. Sex differences in circulating T-tau trajectories after sports-concussion and correlation with outcome. Frontiers in Neurology. 2020;**11**:651

[71] Randall J, Mörtberg E, Provuncher GK, et al. Tau proteins in serum predict neurological outcome after hypoxic brain injury from cardiac arrest:

Results of a pilot study. Resuscitation. 2013;**84**:351-356

[72] Shahim P, Tegner Y, Wilson DH, et al. Blood biomarkers for brain injury in concussed professional ice hockey players. JAMA Neurology. 2014;**71**:684

[73] Shahim P, Tegner Y, Marklund N, Blennow K, Zetterberg H. Neurofilament light and tau as blood biomarkers for sports-related concussion. Neurology. 2018;**90**:E1780-E1788

[74] Gill J, Mustapic M, Diaz-Arrastia R, et al. Higher exosomal tau, amyloid-beta 42 and IL-10 are associated with mild TBIs and chronic symptoms in military personnel. Brain Injury. 2018;**32**:1277-1284

[75] Bogoslovsky T, Wilson D, Chen Y, et al. Increases of plasma levels of glial fibrillary acidic protein, tau, and amyloid β up to 90 days after traumatic brain injury. Journal of Neurotrauma. 2017;**34**:66-73

[76] Liliang PC, Liang CL, Weng HC, et al. τ proteins in serum predict outcome after severe traumatic brain injury. The Journal of Surgical Research. 2010;**160**:302-307

[77] Smith GS, Schneiderman AI, Bailes JE. The epidemiology of sports-related traumatic brain injury. Current Sports Medicine Reports. 2009;**8**:202-207

[78] Guskiewicz KM, Marshall SW, Bailes J, et al. Epidemiology of concussion in collegiate and high school football players. The American Journal of Sports Medicine. 2000;**28**:643-650

[79] Hoge CW, McGurk D, Thomas JL, et al. Mild traumatic brain injury in U.S. soldiers returning from Iraq. The New England Journal of Medicine. 2008;**358**:453-463

[80] Broglio SP, MacKenzie EJ, Sills AK, et al. A systematic review of high school and collegiate American football games: Player injury rate and injury risk per 1,000 athlete-exposures. The American Journal of Sports Medicine. 2009;**37**:519-528

[81] Yang H, Chen Y, Wei L, et al. Increased serum levels of inflammatory biomarkers in patients with mild traumatic brain injury: A systematic review and meta-analysis. Journal of Neurotrauma. 2017;**34**:623-632

[82] Kolls JK, McCray PB Jr. The immune response to respiratory viruses. Nature Reviews. Immunology. 2004;**4**:667-676

[83] Iwamoto T, Iwamoto Y, Masumoto K, et al. Elevated serum levels of cytokines in patients with mild head injury. Brain Injury. 2004;**18**:421-426

[84] Bazarian JJ, Biberthaler P, Welch RD, et al. Serum S100B and neuron-specific enolase and their role as markers of brain injury. Journal of Neurotrauma. 2005;**22**:1457-1465

[85] Killgore WDS, Singh P, Kipman M, Pisner D, Fridman A, Weber M. Gray matter volume and executive functioning correlate with time since injury following mild traumatic brain injury. Neuroscience Letters. 2016;**612**:238-244. DOI: 10.1016/j.neulet.2015.12.033

[86] Motzkin JC, Philippi CL, Wolf RC, Baskaya MK, Koenigs M. Ventromedial prefrontal cortex is critical for the regulation of amygdala activity in humans. Biological Psychiatry. 2015;**77**:276-284. DOI: 10.1016/j.biopsych.2014.02.014

[87] Smits M, Houston GC, Dippel DWJ, Wielopolski PA, Vernooij MW, Koudstaal PJ, et al. Microstructural brain

injury in post-concussion syndrome after minor head injury. Neuroradiology. 2011;**53**:553-563. DOI: 10.1007/s00234-010-0774-6

[88] Messé A, Caplain S, Paradot G, Garrigue D, Mineo JF, Ares GS, et al. Diffusion tensor imaging and white matter lesions at the subacute stage in mild traumatic brain injury with persistent neurobehavioral impairment. Human Brain Mapping. 2011;**32**:999-1011. DOI: 10.1002/hbm.21092

[89] Messé A, Caplain S, Pélégrini-Issac M, Blancho S, Montreuil M, Lévy R, et al. Structural integrity and postconcussion syndrome in mild traumatic brain injury patients. Brain Imaging and Behavior. 2012;**6**:283-292. DOI: 10.1007/s11682-012-9159-2

[90] Yeh PH, Wang B, Oakes TR, French LM, Pan H, Graner J, et al. Postconcussional disorder and PTSD symptoms of military-related traumatic brain injury associated with compromised neurocircuitry. Human Brain Mapping. 2014;**35**:2652-2673. DOI: 10.1002/hbm.22358

[91] Yeh PH, Koay CG, Wang B, Morissette J, Sham E, Senseney J, et al. Compromised neurocircuitry in chronic blast-related mild traumatic brain injury. Human Brain Mapping. 2017;**38**:352-369. DOI: 10.1002/hbm.23365

[92] Delano-Wood L, Bangen KJ, Sorg SF, Clark AL, Schiehser DM, Luc N, et al. Brainstem white matter integrity is related to loss of consciousness and postconcussive symptomatology in veterans with chronic mild to moderate traumatic brain injury. Brain Imaging and Behavior. 2015;**9**:500-512. DOI: 10.1007/s11682-015-9432-2

[93] Rangaprakash D, Deshpande G, Daniel TA, Goodman AM, Robinson JL, Salibi N, et al. Compromised hippocampus-striatum pathway as a potential imaging biomarker of mild-traumatic brain injury and posttraumatic stress disorder. Human Brain Mapping. 2017;**38**:2843-2864. DOI: 10.1002/hbm.23551

[94] Miller DR, Hayes JP, Lafleche G, Salat DH, Verfaellie M. White matter abnormalities are associated with chronic postconcussion symptoms in blast-related mild traumatic brain injury. Human Brain Mapping. 2016;**37**:220-229. DOI: 10.1002/hbm.23022

[95] Egner T, Hirsch J. The neural correlates and functional integration of cognitive control in a stroop task. NeuroImage. 2005;**24**:539-547. DOI: 10.1016/j.neuroimage.2004.09.007

[96] Smits M, Dippel DWJ, Houston GC, Wielopolski PA, Koudstaal PJ, Hunink MGM, et al. Postconcussion syndrome after minor head injury: Brain activation of working memory and attention. Human Brain Mapping. 2009;**30**:2789-2803. DOI: 10.1002/hbm.20709

[97] Owen AM, McMillan KM, Laird AR, Bullmore E. N-back working memory paradigm: A meta-analysis of normative functional neuroimaging studies. Human Brain Mapping. 2005;**25**:46-59. DOI: 10.1002/hbm.20131

[98] Gosselin N, Bottari C, Chen JK, Huntgeburth SC, De Beaumont L, Petrides ML, et al. Evaluating the cognitive consequences of mild traumatic brain injury and concussion by using electrophysiology. Neurosurgical Focus. 2012;**33**(E7):1-7. DOI: 10.3171/2012.10.FOCUS12253

[99] Van der Horn HJ, Liemburg EJ, Scheenen ME, De Koning ME, Spikman JM, Van der Naalt J.

Post-concussive complaints after mild traumatic brain injury associated with altered brain networks during working memory performance. Brain Imaging and Behavior. 2016;**10**:1243-1253. DOI: 10.1007/s11682-015-9489-y

[100] Gosselin N, Bottari C, Chen JK, Petrides M, Tinawi S, De Guise E, et al. Electrophysiology and functional MRI in post-acute mild traumatic brain injury. Journal of Neurotrauma. 2011;**28**:329-341. DOI: 10.1089/neu.2010.1493

[101] Koski L, Kolivakis T, Yu C, Chen JK, Delaney S, Ptito A. Noninvasive brain stimulation for persistent postconcussion symptoms in mild traumatic brain injury. Journal of Neurotrauma. 2015;**32**:38-44. DOI: 10.1089/neu.2014.3449

[102] Astafiev SV, Zinn KL, Shulman GL, Corbetta M. Exploring the physiological correlates of chronic mild traumatic brain injury symptoms. NeuroImage: Clinical. 2016;**11**:10-19. DOI: 10.1016/j.nicl.2016.01.004

[103] Stevens MC, Lovejoy D, Kim J, Oakes H, Kureshi I, Witt ST. Multiple resting state network functional connectivity abnormalities in mild traumatic brain injury. Brain Imaging and Behavior. 2012;**6**:293-318. DOI: 10.1007/s11682-012-9157-4

[104] Kaushal M, España LY, Nencka AS, Wang Y, Nelson LD, McCrea MA, et al. Resting-state functional connectivity after concussion is associated with clinical recovery. Human Brain Mapping. 2019;**40**:1211-1220. DOI: 10.1002/hbm.24440

[105] Palacios EM, Yuh EL, Chang YS, Yue JK, Schnyer DM, Okonkwo DO, et al. Resting-state functional connectivity alterations associated with six-month outcomes in mild traumatic brain injury. Journal of Neurotrauma. 2017;**34**:1546-1557. DOI: 10.1089/neu.2016.4752

[106] Zhou Y, Milham MP, Lui YW, Miles L, Reaume J, Sodickson DK, et al. Default-mode network disruption in mild traumatic brain injury. Radiology. 2012;**265**:882-892. DOI: 10.1148/radiol.12120748

[107] Vanhaudenhuyse A, Demertzi A, Schabus M, Noirhomme Q, Bredart S, Boly M, et al. Two distinct neuronal networks mediate the awareness of environment and of self. Journal of Cognitive Neuroscience. 2011;**23**:570-578. DOI: 10.1162/jocn.2010.21488

[108] Sours C, Chen H, Roys S, Zhuo J, Varshney A, Gullapalli RP. Investigation of multiple frequency ranges using discrete wavelet decomposition of resting-state functional connectivity in mild traumatic brain injury patients. Brain Connectivity. 2015;**5**:442-450. DOI: 10.1089/brain.2014.0333

[109] Zhou Y. Small world properties changes in mild traumatic brain injury. Journal of Magnetic Resonance Imaging. 2017;**46**:518-527. DOI: 10.1002/jmri.25548

[110] Van der Werf YD, Witter MP, Uylings HBM, Jolles J. Neuropsychology of infarctions in the thalamus: A review. Neuropsychologia. 2000;**38**:613-627. DOI: 10.1016/S0028-3932(99)00104-9

[111] Messé A, Caplain S, Pélégrini-Issac M, Blancho S, Lévy R, Aghakhani N, et al. Specific and evolving resting-state network alterations in post-concussion syndrome following mild traumatic brain injury. PLoS One. 2013;**8**:e65470. DOI: 10.1371/journal.pone.0065470

[112] Chong CD, Wang L, Wang K, Traub S, Li J. Homotopic region

connectivity during concussion recovery: A longitudinal fMRI study. PLoS One. 2019;**14**:e0221892. DOI: 10.1371/journal.pone.0221892

[113] Oliver JM, Jones MT, Kirk KM, Gable DA, Repshas JT, Johnson TA, et al. Serum Neurofilament light in American football athletes over the course of a season. Journal of Neurotrauma. 2016;**33**:1784-1789. DOI: 10.1089/neu.2015.4295

[114] Zetterberg H, Tanriverdi F, Unluhizarci K, Selcuklu A, Kelestimur F, Blennow K. Sustained release of neuron-specific enolase to serum in amateur boxers. Brain Injury. 2009;**23**:723-726. DOI: 10.1080/02699050903120399

[115] McMahon PJ, Panczykowski DM, Yue JK, Puccio AM, Inoue T, Sorani MD, et al. Measurement of the glial fibrillary acidic protein and its breakdown products GFAP-BDP biomarker for the detection of traumatic brain injury compared to computed tomography and magnetic resonance imaging. Journal of Neurotrauma. 2015;**32**:527-533. DOI: 10.1089/neu.2014.3635

[116] Stein DM, Lindell A, Murdock KR, Kufera JA, Menaker J, Keledjian K, et al. Relationship of serum and cerebrospinal fluid biomarkers with intracranial hypertension and cerebral hypoperfusion after severe traumatic brain injury. The Journal of Trauma. 2011;**70**:1096-1103. DOI: 10.1097/TA.0b013e318216930d

[117] Shahim P, Tegner Y, Marklund N, Höglund K, Portelius E, Brody DL, et al. Astroglial activation and altered amyloid metabolism in human repetitive concussion. Neurology. 2017;**88**:1400-1407. DOI: 10.1212/WNL.0000000000003816

[118] Shahim P, Tegner Y, Gustafsson B, Gren M, Ärlig J, Olsson M, et al. Neurochemical aftermath of repetitive mild traumatic brain injury. JAMA Neurology. 2016;**73**:1308-1315. DOI: 10.1001/jamaneurol.2016.2038

[119] Alosco ML, Tripodis Y, Fritts NG, Heslegrave A, Baugh CM, Conneely S, et al. Cerebrospinal fluid tau, Aβ, and sTREM2 in former National Football League players: Modelling the relationship between repetitive head impacts, microglial activation, and neurodegeneration. Alzheimer's & Dementia. 2018;**14**:1159-1170. DOI: 10.1016/j.jalz.2018.05.004

[120] Singhal A, Baker AJ, Hare GMT, Reinders FX, Schlichter LC, Moulton RJ. Association between cerebrospinal fluid Interleukin-6 concentrations and outcome after severe human traumatic brain injury. Journal of Neurotrauma. 2002;**19**:929-937. DOI: 10.1089/089771502320317087

[121] Yoshizawa JM, Schafer CA, Schafer JJ, Farrell JJ, Paster BJ, Wong DTW. Salivary biomarkers: Toward future clinical and diagnostic utilities. Clinical Microbiology Reviews. 2013;**26**:781-791

[122] Kaufman E, Lamster IB. The diagnostic applications of saliva—A review. Critical Reviews in Oral Biology and Medicine. 2002;**13**:197-212

[123] Dhima M, Salinas TJ, Wermers RA, Weaver AL, Koka S. Preference changes of adult outpatients for giving saliva, urine and blood for clinical testing after actual sample collection. Journal of Prosthodontic Research. 2013;**57**:51-56

[124] Abraham JE, Maranian MJ, Spiteri I, Russell R, Ingle S, Luccarini C, et al. Saliva samples are a viable alternative to blood samples as a source of DNA for high throughput genotyping. BMC Medical Genomics. 2012;**5**:19

[125] Melguizo-Rodríguez L, Costela-Ruiz V, Manzano-Moreno F, Ruiz C, Illescas-Montes R. Salivary biomarkers and their application in the diagnosis and monitoring of the Most common Oral pathologies. International Journal of Molecular Sciences. 2020;**21**:5173

[126] Salazar-Ruales C, Arguello J-V, López-Cortés A, Cabrera-Andrade A, García-Cárdenas JM, Guevara-Ramírez P, et al. Salivary MicroRNAs for early detection of head and neck squamous cell carcinoma: A case-control study in the high altitude mestizo Ecuadorian population. BioMed Research International. 2018;**2018**:9792730

[127] Dadas A, Washington J, Diaz-Arrastia R, Janigro D. Biomarkers in traumatic brain injury (TBI): A review. Neuropsychiatric Disease and Treatment. 2018;**14**:2989-3000

[128] Hier DB, Obafemi-Ajayi T, Thimgan MS, Olbricht GR, Azizi S, Allen B, et al. Blood biomarkers for mild traumatic brain injury: A selective review of unresolved issues. Biomarker Research. 2021;**9**:70

[129] Zhang J, Puvenna V, Janigro D. Biomarkers of traumatic brain injury and their relationship to pathology. In: Laskowitz D, Grant G, editors. Translational Research in Traumatic Brain Injury. Boca Raton, FL, USA: CRC Press/Taylor and Francis Group; 2016; Chapter 12

[130] Dadas A, Janigro D. The role and diagnostic significance of cellular barriers after concussive head trauma. Concussion. 2018;**3**:CNC53

[131] Murcko R, Marchi N, Bailey D, Janigro D. Diagnostic biomarker kinetics: How brain-derived biomarkers distribute through the human body, and how this affects their diagnostic significance: The case of S100B. Fluids and Barriers of the CNS. 2022;**19**:32

[132] Donato R. Intracellular and extracellular roles of S100 proteins. Microscopy Research and Technique. 2003;**60**:540-551

[133] Chong Z, Changyaleket B, Xu H, Dull R, Schwartz D. Identifying S100B as a biomarker and a therapeutic target for brain injury and multiple diseases. Current Medicinal Chemistry. 2016;**23**:1571-1596

[134] Janigro D, Kawata K, Silverman E, Marchi N, Diaz-Arrastia R. Is salivary S100B a biomarker of traumatic brain injury? A pilot study. Frontiers in Neurology. 2020;**11**:528

[135] Yeung C, Bhatia R, Bhattarai B, Sinha M. Role of salivary biomarkers in predicting significant traumatic brain injury: An exploratory study. Pediatric Emergency Care. 2020;**37**:e1373-e1376

[136] Monroe DC, Thomas EA, Cecchi NJ, Granger DA, Hicks JW, Small SL. Salivary S100 calcium-binding protein beta (S100B) and neurofilament light (NfL) after acute exposure to repeated head impacts in collegiate water polo players. Scientific Reports. 2022;**12**:3439

[137] Abu-Rumeileh S, Abdelhak A, Foschi M, D'Anna L, Russo M, Steinacker P, et al. The multifaceted role of neurofilament light chain protein in non-primary neurological diseases. Brain. 2022;**146**:421-437

[138] Gaetani L, Blennow K, Calabresi P, Di Filippo M, Parnetti L, Zetterberg H. Neurofilament light chain as a biomarker in neurological disorders. Journal of Neurology, Neurosurgery, and Psychiatry. 2019;**90**:870-881

[139] Thebault S, Booth R, Freedman M. Blood Neurofilament light chain: The Neurologist's troponin? Biomedicine. 2020;**8**:523

[140] Karantali E, Kazis D, McKenna J, Chatzikonstantinou S, Petridis F, Mavroudis I. Neurofilament light chain in patients with a concussion or head impacts: A systematic review and meta-analysis. European Journal of Trauma and Emergency Surgery. 2021;**48**:1555-1567

[141] Hiskens MI, Mengistu TS, Li KM, Fenning AS. Systematic review of the diagnostic and clinical utility of salivary microRNAs in traumatic brain injury (TBI). International Journal of Molecular Sciences. 2022;**23**:13160

[142] Johnson JJ, Loeffert AC, Stokes J, Olympia RP, Bramley H, Hicks SD. Association of Salivary MicroRNA changes with prolonged concussion symptoms. JAMA Pediatrics. 2018;**172**:65-73

[143] LaRocca D, Barns S, Hicks SD, Brindle A, Williams J, Uhlig R, et al. Comparison of serum and saliva miRNAs for identification and characterization of mTBI in adult mixed martial arts fighters. PLoS One. 2019;**14**:e0207785

[144] Hicks SD, Onks C, Kim RY, Zhen KJ, Loeffert J, Loeffert AC, et al. Diagnosing mild traumatic brain injury using saliva RNA compared to cognitive and balance testing. Clinical and Translational Medicine. 2020;**10**:e197

[145] Di Pietro V, O'Halloran P, Watson CN, Begum G, Acharjee A, Yakoub KM, et al. Unique diagnostic signatures of concussion in the saliva of male athletes: The study of concussion in Rugby union through MicroRNAs (SCRUM). British Journal of Sports Medicine. 2021;**55**:1395-1404

[146] Fedorchak G, Rangnekar A, Onks C, Loeffert AC, Loeffert J, Olympia RP, et al. Saliva RNA biomarkers predict concussion duration and detect symptom recovery: A comparison with balance and cognitive testing. Journal of Neurology. 2021;**268**:4349-4361

[147] Khan NA, Asim M, El-Menyar A, Biswas KH, Rizoli S, Al-Thani H. The evolving role of extracellular vesicles (exosomes) as biomarkers in traumatic brain injury: Clinical perspectives and therapeutic implications. Frontiers in Aging Neuroscience. 2022;**14**:933434

[148] Hill AF. Extracellular vesicles and neurodegenerative diseases. The Journal of Neuroscience. 2019;**39**:9269-9273

[149] Cheng Y, Pereira M, Raukar N, Reagan JL, Queseneberry M, Goldberg L, et al. Potential biomarkers to detect traumatic brain injury by the profiling of salivary extracellular vesicles. Journal of Cellular Physiology. 2019;**234**:14377-14388

[150] Matuk R, Pereira M, Baird J, Dooner M, Cheng Y, Wen S, et al. The role of salivary vesicles as a potential inflammatory biomarker to detect traumatic brain injury in mixed martial artists. Scientific Reports. 2021;**11**:8186

Chapter 6

The Ferroptosis in Traumatic Brain Injury: The Future Direction?

Lifeng Qian, Sunfeng Pan, Yanbing Feng, Hanqiang Shi, Lie Xiong, Fuxiang Zhu, Yanbo Shi and Zhongwei Yu

Abstract

Traumatic brain injury (TBI) is a severe acute brain injury caused by external mechanical force, resulting in temporary or permanent impairment of physical, psychological, cognitive functions, and altered consciousness states. Cognitive dysfunction commonly leading to symptoms such as inattention and decline in learning and memory abilities, and may also result in irritability, anxiety or depression. The underlying pathology involves significant neuron loss and limited synaptic remodeling. Abnormal iron metabolism is common in the brains of patients with TBI and cognitive impairment. However, effective intervention measures are still lacking which prompts us to explore new therapeutic targets and develop novel therapies for TBI. As a newly discovered form of regulated cell death, ferroptosis occurs due to excessive iron accumulation in the brain, leading to cellular and neuronal damage. Iron overload and ferroptosis play a significant role in the pathophysiology of secondary brain injury. Therefore, potential therapeutic approaches may involve targeting factors such as iron deposition and ferroptosis inhibition. This chapter provides an overview of ferroptosis' role in traumatic brain injury (TBI) and advance investigation in related research fields with the aim of enhancing our understanding of TBI treatment through ferroptosis inhibition, ultimately guiding new clinical directions for further TBI research.

Keywords: traumatic brain injury, ferroptosis, iron metabolic disorder, iron chelator, reactive oxygen species, blood-brain barrier

1. Introduction

Traumatic brain injury (TBI) is a frequently occurring disease resulting from injuries in the emergency department. It is also a leading cause of disability and paralysis worldwide among trauma-related injuries. According to statistics, approximately 50 million individuals suffer from varying degrees of TBI annually. The primary causes of TBI include traffic accidents, falls from heights, violent attacks, slips and falls. In addition to direct trauma-induced injury, patients typically experience severe neuronal necrosis, brain tissue edema, disruption of the blood-brain barrier (BBB), heightened oxidative stress, and excessive inflammation following TBI. Several factors mechanistically contribute to secondary injury including excitability,

IntechOpen

mitochondrial dysfunction, oxidative stress, lipid peroxidation neuroinflammation, axonal degeneration, and apoptotic cell death (**Figure 1**).

These factors result in consequences such as disruption of the blood-brain barrier (BBB), release of blood metabolites, activation of microglia, thrombin activity, excitatory amino acids, and proinflammatory cytokines (**Figure 1**). This creates a harmful cycle [1]. Patients with varying degrees of traumatic brain injury (TBI) may experience different levels of secondary damage [2]. Some evidence suggests an increased occurrence of neurodegenerative diseases like Alzheimer's disease, Parkinson's disease, and chronic traumatic encephalopathy caused by head trauma. Treatment for TBI may involve options such as pharmacotherapy, cognitive therapy, or surgery. There is a growing demand for agents that can potentially alleviate primary brain injury aspects and mitigate the secondary pathological deficits associated with TBI.

In recent years, several studies have indicated that abnormal iron metabolism is prevalent in the brains of patients with traumatic brain injury and cognitive impairment. Furthermore, an increase in brain iron content has been linked to cognitive decline. Iron, as an essential trace element for maintaining normal physiological functions in the human body, plays a crucial role in various aspects such as electron transport, cell respiration, and DNA synthesis. However, like everything else, iron also has its drawbacks and can be a "double-edged sword." Its balanced metabolism is vital for sustaining overall bodily function; any imbalance can lead to a range of diseases. Studies on chronic traumatic encephalopathy have revealed that tau overdeposition and neurofibrillary tangle formation are typical pathological features observed during autopsies [3, 4]. Excessive deposition of iron has also been found within these neurofibrillary tangles where oxidative stress-induced phosphorylation of tau occurs [5, 6]. Interestingly, earlier reports demonstrated non-heme iron deposition in the deep cortex and hippocampus of postmortem brain tissue from mTBI patients [5]. Consequently, iron has gradually emerged as a potential target for intervention in TBI research. Therefore, it is believed that imbalances in iron homeostasis play a significant role in influencing the pathological processes associated with TBI.

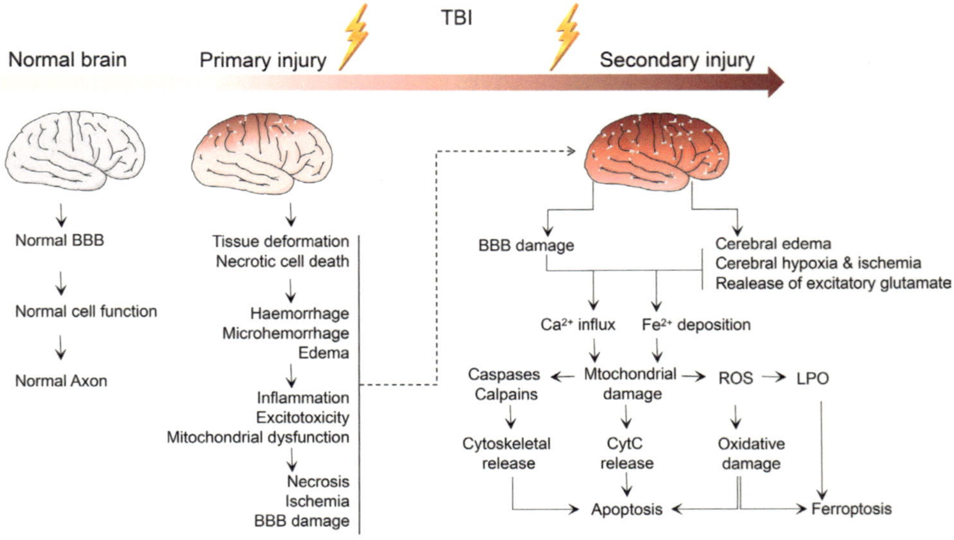

Figure 1.
The pathophysiological mechanism of primary and secondary brain injury.

Iron is the most abundant metal trace element in the brain and plays a crucial role in the development of the central nervous system (CNS), contributing to the synthesis of myelin and various neurotransmitters [7, 8]. Insufficient iron levels during lactation can impair neurotransmitter synthesis, leading to developmental disorders in behavioral functions. Conversely, excessive intracellular iron can disrupt neurological function, particularly in brains affected by traumatic brain injury (TBI). TBI-induced damage to brain tissue, disruption of the blood-brain barrier, increased cerebral vascular permeability, and severe local inflammatory reactions result in an influx of iron from the bloodstream into the brain parenchyma. Neuronal death is one of the most serious consequences following TBI.

Ferroptosis is a newly discovered mode of cell death characterized by iron-dependent lipid peroxidation. Specifically, excess iron, in the form of divalent ferrous ion Fe^{2+}, can react with hydrogen peroxide (H_2O_2) or organic hydrogen peroxide (ROOH) to produce soluble hydroxyl (HO) or lipid alkoxy (RO•) groups, respectively. These reactions are the main source of reactive oxygen species (ROS), known as the Fenton reaction [9], which ultimately leads to cell death. Neurons, being terminally differentiated cells, experience various cellular stresses throughout their lifespan. Oxidative stress is one of the key ones, which is caused by excessive accumulation of intracellular ROS. Neuronal membranes contain high levels of cholesterol and polyunsaturated fatty acids (PUFAs), making them susceptible to oxidation by ROS and resulting in oxidative damage [10]. Additionally, neurons have limited ability to scavenge ROS autonomously due to relatively low levels of antioxidant factors such as superoxide dismutase (SOD) and glutathione peroxidase (GPX) compared to other tissues in the brain [11, 12]. The aforementioned evidence further supports the notion that neurons are particularly vulnerable to iron overload. These findings have led researchers to speculate that ferroptosis may play a significant role in cognitive dysfunction resulting from traumatic brain injury (TBI). Furthermore, recent studies have indeed demonstrated activation of the ferroptosis pathway after TBI leading to neuronal death.

The aforementioned studies all indicate a strong correlation between disrupted iron homeostasis and unfavorable prognosis in patients with traumatic brain injury (TBI). In this chapter, we aim to delve into the role of iron and ferroptosis in brain injuries, enhance our comprehension of iron metabolism and the significance of ferroptosis in TBI, as well as explore novel effective treatment approaches for managing iron dysregulation and ferroptosis following TBI.

2. Brain iron metabolism

Iron is the most abundant trace element in the brain and is crucial for brain development and proper functioning. Iron can be found in various components of the brain, including neurons, astrocytes, oligodendrocytes, axons, microglia, and myelin [7, 13, 14]. It plays a vital role in processes such as myelination, neuroectoderm development, oxygen transport, neurotransmitter transmission, and mitochondrial energy production [8, 15].

To reach the CNS, iron must pass through either the blood-brain barrier or the blood-CSF-brain (BCSF) and be taken up by brain tissue cells. The blood-brain barrier is crucial in protecting the brain from fluctuations in systemic iron levels and plays a vital role in brain iron uptake. Iron enters capillary epithelial cells of brain tissue via endocytosis, with Fe^{2+} most likely transported out by Fpn1. Similar cells include BBB endothelial cells, neural tube cells, oligodendrocytes, astrocytes, choroid plexus cells, and ependymal cells.

Iron in the bloodstream enters the brain through the blood-brain barrier in two main forms: the transferrin-bound iron-transferrin receptor complex and non-transferrin-bound iron [16].

Studies have reported that endothelial cells in the choroid plexus also play a role in regulating iron entry into the central nervous system [17]. Astrocytes facilitate the redistribution of iron within the central nervous system with the assistance of ceruloplasmin, which has already crossed the blood-brain barrier to other cells [13]. Ceruloplasmin oxidizes divalent iron to Fe^{3+}, which then binds to transferrin and enters the cerebrospinal fluid (CSF) [16].

In addition, in cells that do not express the transferrin receptor, significant amounts of non-transferrin binding iron circulate in the cerebrospinal fluid (CSF) along with ATP, citrate, and ascorbic acid [7, 18]. Oligodendrocytes possess the highest iron content in the brain [19], which may explain their heightened susceptibility to oxidative stress [20]. While oligodendrocytes are primarily responsible for expressing and secreting transferrin, they also uptake non-transferrin-bound iron through Tim-2 receptors via ferritin. Astrocytes acquire non-transferrin-bound iron through DMT1 uptake [17, 21–23]. Neurons obtain iron from CSF and interstitial fluid by binding it to transferrin.

Lactoferrin [24] and its receptor, lactoferrin receptor (LfR), as well as glycosyl phosphatidylinositol (GPI)-anchored melanotransferrin (MTf) and secreted melanotransferrin, may also contribute to the transportation of iron across the blood-brain barrier [25, 26].

At acidic pH, trivalent iron (Fe^{3+}) is released from endosomes and subsequently reduced to divalent iron (Fe^{2+}). Divalent metal transporter 1 (DMT1, also known as SLC11A2) facilitates the release of Fe^{2+} from endosomes into unstable iron stores in the cytoplasm [7]. Ceruloplasmin is a GPI-linked membrane protein expressed mainly in astrocytes surrounding brain microvessels within the mammalian central nervous system [27]. Following the discovery of ceruloplasmin's ferroxidase activity, it was suggested that its role in iron metabolism involves aiding the cellular export of iron by binding to membrane ferroportin [28, 29].

Abnormalities in iron metabolism, including both iron deficiency and iron overload, have a negative impact on overall bodily functions and are associated with various diseases. Iron deficiency specifically reduces cytochrome oxidase activity in the brain, particularly in the hippocampus and prefrontal regions [30], potentially leading to disorders in brain development such as motor skills and cognitive memory [31]. Conversely, excessive levels of iron can accumulate in the brain and contribute to neurodegenerative diseases like Parkinson's disease (PD) and Alzheimer's disease (AD) [32, 33]. Additionally, neuroferritinopathies associated with traumatic brain injury (TBI) have also been identified as neurodegenerative conditions characterized by abnormal iron accumulation [34].

3. Ferroptosis and its regulation

3.1 Ferroptosis is a new type of iron-dependent cell death

Ferroptosis is a new mode of cell death discovered by Stockwell's group at Columbia University in the past decade [9]. When they observed that the small molecule compound Erastin killed RAS mutant tumor cells, they found that the death mode was different from apoptosis, necrosis or autophagy, etc., but it could be effectively inhibited by the iron chelator deferoxamine (DFO), so they named this iron-dependent cell death ferroptosis [35, 36].

3.2 The regulatory mechanism of ferroptosis is complex

With the deepening of research, scientists have found that there is a complex and fine regulatory network of ferroptosis, including inhibition of ferroptosis pathway and activation of ferroptosis pathway (**Figure 2**).

3.2.1 Inhibition of ferroptosis pathway

The regulatory system of GPX4, along with the GPX4-independent resistance ferroptosis pathway, are included in these mechanisms.

(1) The GSH-GPX4 antioxidant system in the cytoplasm and mitochondria is an important pathway for cells to defend against ferroptosis. The cystine/glutamate antiporter (SLC7A11/SLC3A2, also known as System Xc^-) on the cell membrane transports cystine into the cell and releases glutamate into the extracellular space at a 1:1 ratio [31]. Once inside the cell, cystine can be converted to cysteine, which is further processed by glutamate cysteine ligase (GCL) and glutathione synthetase (GSS). The reduced form of nicotinamide adenine dinucleotide phosphate (NADPH) serves as an important reducing agent for synthesizing Glutathione (GSH). By utilizing GSH as a reducing cofactor, lipid peroxidases are ultimately converted to lipid alcohols by cytoplasmic and mitochondrial glutathione peroxidase GPX4 [37].

(2) The GPX4-independent pathway of ferroptosis resistance involves the FSP1-CoQ_{10} pathway, a cell membrane-based inhibitor that prevents lipid peroxide

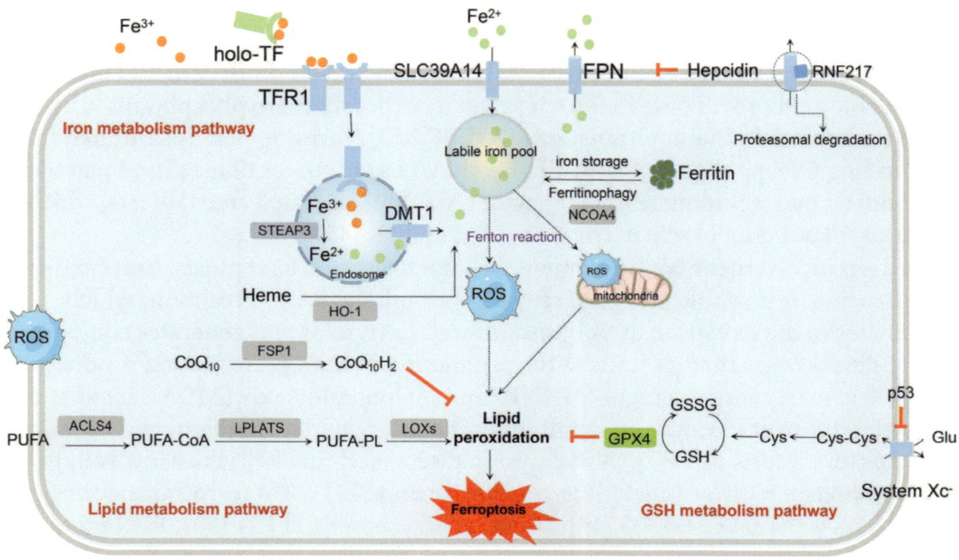

Figure 2.
Molecular mechanism of ferroptosis.

generation by trapping lipophilic free radicals. Myristoylated FSP1 (also known as apoptosis-inducing factor mitochondrial 2, AIFM2) acts as an oxidorereductase of CoQ_{10} at the plasma membrane and plays a crucial role in this process [38, 39].

(3) GPX4-independent ferroptosis resistance pathway, GTP cyclohydrogenase 1-tetrahydrobiopterin (GCH1-BH4) pathway in cytoplasm. GCH1 and its metabolic derivative, tetrahydrobiopterin/dihydrobiopterin (BH4/BH2), protect against ferrodeath by selectively inhibiting the depletion of phospholipids containing two polyunsaturated fatty acyl groups [40, 41].

(4) GPX4-independent ferroptosis resistance pathway, known as the dihydroorotate dehydrogenase (DHODH-$CoQ_{10}H_2$) pathway in mitochondria, plays a crucial role in protecting against ferroptosis. Dihydroorotate dehydrogenase (DHODH), an enzyme dependent on flavin, is located in the inner mitochondrial membrane and primarily functions to catalyze the fourth step of pyrimidine biosynthesis. During this process, dihydroorotate (DHO) is oxidized to orotate (OA), while simultaneously transferring electrons to ubiquinone in the mitochondrial inner membrane. This leads to the reduction of ubiquinone into dihydroubiquinone ($CoQ_{10}H_2$), which contributes to mitigating ferroptosis within mitochondria. Furthermore, it was found that DHODH inhibits lipid peroxidation and suppresses ferroptosis within mitochondria when GPX4 expression is low. However, under conditions of high GPX4 expression, a combination of ferroptosis inducers such as sulfasalazine and DHODH inhibitors can activate ferroptosis [42].

3.2.2 Activation of ferroptosis pathway

Lipid peroxidation is the main driver of ferroptosis. Intracellular accumulation of free fatty acids is induced by acetyl-CoA carboxylase (ACAC)-mediated fatty acid synthesis or lipophagy-mediated fatty acid release, ultimately leading to ferroptosis [43]. Acyl-coa synthetase long-chain family member 4 (ACSL4) connects polyunsaturated fatty acids (PUFAs), including arachidonic acid and docosatetraenoic acid [44]. These PUFAs are then incorporated into phospholipids by lysophosphatidylcholine acyltransferase 3 (LPCAT3), forming polyunsaturated fatty acid binding phospholipids (PUFA-PLs). PUFA-PLs are susceptible to lipid peroxidation induced by arachidonate lipoxygenase (ALOXs)-mediated free radicals, which ultimately play a crucial role in triggering ferroptosis [45].

Iron ion involvement is a fundamental characteristic of ferroptosis. Iron catalyzes the formation of unstable hydroxyl radicals through the Fenton reaction, which participates in the oxidation of polyunsaturated fatty acids and generates conjugated dienes. This process further leads to the production of lipid peroxidation products such as 4-hydroxynonenoic acid (4-HNE) and malondialdehyde (MDA). It enhances the vulnerability of various cell membranes, impairs cellular function, and ultimately promotes ferroptosis [46, 47]. Wang's group discovered that key genes involved in iron metabolism pathway, including transferrin and SLC39A14 ferrotransporter [48], ferritin heavy chain (FTH) [35, 49], transferrin receptor (TFR1) [50], FPN pump ferritin [51, 52], iron chaperone binding protein (PCBP1), [53], and nuclear receptor coactivator 4(NCOA4) [54, 55] reported by other research groups have been found to regulate ferroptosis by controlling iron metabolism. It is evident that understanding the biological role of iron and its metabolic pathways in ferroptosis is crucial; therefore, further exploration into underlying mechanisms is necessary.

4. The roles of iron and ferroptosis in TBI

4.1 Imbalance of iron homeostasis in TBI

Studies have confirmed that iron homeostasis in the brain is disrupted following TBI (**Figure 3**). Several potential causes include abnormal iron deposition due to erythrocyte lysis, mitochondrial and lysosomal dysfunction, and regulatory effects on iron metabolism networks.

TBI encompasses both primary and secondary impairments. Primary injury refers to fractures of the head caused by external forces, resulting in cortical or subcortical contusions and lacerations, intracranial hemorrhage (subarachnoid hemorrhage or subdural hematoma), and disruption of the blood-brain barrier (BBB). Diffuse axonal injury (DAI), which is the hallmark injury of TBI, is primarily responsible for long-term complications that may arise from a combination of neuroinflammation and neurodegeneration [56]. Following trauma, axons in the brain's white matter are particularly vulnerable to damage. The main effects of DAI include mechanical rupture of the axonal cytoskeleton, leading to disrupted axonal transport, resulting in swelling and proteolysis within the axons themselves [57]. Secondary injury refers to subsequent molecular and chemical inflammatory reactions such as release of blood hemoglobin and iron, dysfunction in brain metabolism and cerebral blood flow, further triggering processes related to neuroinflammation, oxidative stress, glutamatergic excitotoxicity, mitochondrial dysfunction, etc., all contributing to additional damage within the brain [58].

Some studies have reported intracerebral iron deposition in TBI patients due to the release of heme iron from intracranial hemorrhage. As brain-specific phagocytes, microglia phagocytose red blood cells and then release degraded iron into the brain

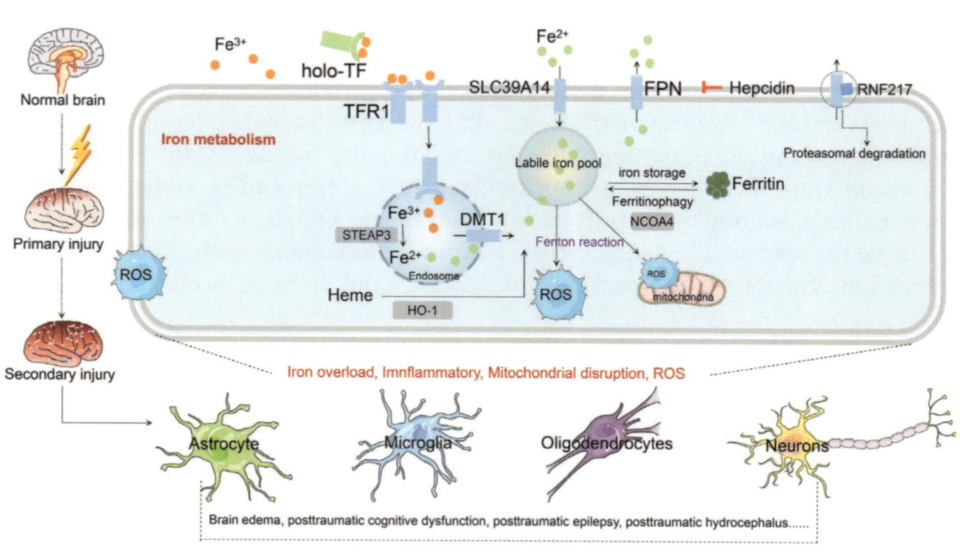

Figure 3.
Imbalance of iron homeostasis in TBI.

interstitium [59]. These mechanisms contribute to an excess accumulation of iron in nerve cells after TBI. The increased levels of iron in both the interstitium and cerebrospinal fluid can be transported to various types of nerve cells through different pathways, ultimately leading to oxidative stress and exacerbating secondary injury following TBI [60].

Iron homeostasis is a dynamic equilibrium regulated by a dynamic network of multiple genes. Following intracerebral hemorrhage, there is an increase in the expression of ferritin, transferrin, and transferrin receptors in the brain, facilitating iron uptake by neurons and oligodendrocytes. Excess Fe can suppress the expression of IRPs in cells and then regulate the increase of ferritin and Fpn1 expression to enhance the capacity of iron pool storage and iron efflux [31, 61]. In patients with TBI, microglia are activated and release toxic substances such as proinflammatory cytokines interleukin (IL-6) and tumor necrosis factor α (TNF-α), complement proteins, and proteases, which contribute to brain injury [62]. With the destruction of the blood-brain barrier and the increase of permeability after TBI, neutrophils and macrophages further infiltrate into the brain tissue [63–65]. They participate in autophagy, secrete anti-inflammatory factors, enhance the clearance of damaged cells, and reduce the toxic effects caused by cellular degradation. Additionally, they promote cellular repair and restore neural plasticity. However, hepcidin expression also increases during inflammation and iron overload in cells [66]. Studies have indicated that hepcidin has the ability to cross the blood-brain barrier and enter the central nervous system [67]. When the blood-brain barrier is compromised, a significant amount of hepcidin can enter brain tissue. The weakened ability of iron efflux further exacerbates the excessive accumulation of iron, resulting in increased production of toxic free radicals and reactive oxygen species (ROS) such as superoxide free radicals and nitric oxide. This ultimately leads to cognitive dysfunction, brain edema, and other detrimental effects. In addition to ROS generation, it also impairs mitochondrial function, reduces mitochondrial respiration, causes lipid peroxidation, and disrupts protein and enzyme oxidation processes, all contributing to neuronal damage [68]. The increased toxicity of extracellular glutamate and the over-stimulation of glutamate N-methyl-D-aspartate (NMDA) and a-amino-3-hydroxy-5-methyl-4-isoxazole-propionic acid receptors can affect calcium uptake, leading to neuronal damage and cell death [69]. Patients with TBI exhibit elevated levels of extracellular glutamate in the cortex and hippocampus, along with reduced glutamate transporters. These alterations result in decreased gabaergic control and heightened epileptic activity, ultimately causing cell death and affecting cognition in a mouse TBI model [70, 71]. At the same time, it can result in mitochondrial dysfunction and excessive production of free radicals, leading to the activation of the caspase signaling pathway and promoting cell apoptosis. The characteristic features of ferroptosis such as mitochondrial destruction, iron deposition, and accumulation of lipid ROS can be observed [72].

4.2 Iron-related brain injury after TBI

4.2.1 Brain edema after trauma

Brain edema after traumatic brain injury (TBI) is the most common and important pathophysiological reaction, which can lead to increased intracranial pressure (ICP) and even lead to brain tissue displacement and herniation. It is a major cause of clinical death and severe disability, with approximately 50% of TBI patients dying from cerebral edema and its associated lesions [73–76]. Typically, brain edema peaks within 2 to 3 days after TBI. Eliminating brain edema has become a key target for the treatment of TBI, which is directly related to the prognosis of patients with traumatic brain injury.

There are two main types of brain edema after TBI, including vasogenic edema and cytotoxic edema. Vasogenic edema is caused by fluid and protein leaking into the brain tissue space due to increased capillary permeability after damage to the blood-brain barrier (BBB), resulting in edema around the brain tissue, which can be seen as a widening of the intercellular space. Cytotoxic edema is caused by an increase in intracellular osmoactive substances, usually due to ion pump dysfunction or subsequent entry of extracellular hypotonic fluid into cells, leading to cell edema. Therefore, cytotoxic edema does not lead to an increase in ICP because it refers only to an increase in intracellular water without a change in overall brain water content [77]. This type of edema occurs in all cell types but mainly results in astrocyte cell edema during the acute phase of TBI. The mechanism of traumatic brain edema is still not fully understood. So far, it is believed that the occurrence and development of traumatic brain edema involve a variety of mechanisms, including blood-brain barrier destruction, Ca^{2+} overload, oxygen-free radical toxicity, cerebral microcirculation disorders, energy metabolism disorders, neurotransmitter toxicity, cytokine release, and autonomic nervous dysfunction.

Recent studies have shown that ferroptosis is also involved in TBI, and ferroptosis inhibitor Ferrostatin-1 can mitigate the levels of IL-1b and TNF-a levels as well as the destruction of BBB, thereby reducing brain edema [78]. At the same time, TBI can disrupt the balance between oxidative and antioxidant systems, potentially leading to brain edema [79]. A decrease in GPX4 is a characteristic marker of ferroptosis occurrence, which is caused by the increase of ROS. In animal models of TBI, overexpression of GPX4 reduced brain edema and blood-brain barrier disruption [78]. PUFAs such as arachidonic acid increase the amount of ROS, leading to ferroptosis. An increase in AA and polyunsaturated fatty acids in the brain leads to an elevation in water and sodium levels, while causing a reduction in potassium and ATP-dependent NaC/KC pumps; consequently, this leads to the development of brain edema [80].

4.2.2 Posttraumatic cognitive dysfunction

Posttraumatic cognitive dysfunction primarily presents as disturbance of consciousness, memory, attention, and learning and processing abilities [81, 82], significantly impacting the patients' quality of life. Individuals with mild TBI may experience temporary disruptions in consciousness, mild confusion, lack of focus, and amnesia immediately following the injury; however, most recover within 6 months [83], with a favorable long-term prognosis. Only a small percentage of individuals with mild TBI will suffer from persistent cognitive impairments [84]. Patients with moderate or severe TBI endure the loss of consciousness for more than 30 minutes or posttraumatic amnesia lasting over 24 hours [85].

Currently, the etiology of cognitive dysfunction remains inconclusive; however, research has postulated the involvement of ferroptosis, diffuse axonal injury (DAI), neuronal abnormalities, and blood-brain barrier (BBB) disruption in this process. Studies have demonstrated reduced levels of glutathione in patients with traumatic brain injury (TBI) [86], as well as iron deposition, which may be associated with cognitive impairment [87]. Intraventricular administration of ferrostatin-1 in animal models of TBI has shown a significant reduction in iron deposition and neuronal degeneration along with improved cognitive function, suggesting a potential role for ferroptosis in the pathogenesis of cognitive impairment [88]. Many studies have demonstrated that head injury is a risk factor for Alzheimer's disease (AD) [89]. The primary characteristic of AD patients is cognitive impairment. Neuronal deficits in AD patients, particularly hippocampal neuronal damage accompanied by increased ferroptosis, suggest the activation of the Nrf2/GPX4 signaling pathway, which may also contribute to cognitive impairment in traumatic brain injury (TBI) patients [90, 91]. Animal models of AD have indicated that blood-brain barrier (BBB) damage occurs early in the course of the disease [92]. Therefore, BBB impairment in TBI patients may also play a role in cognitive dysfunction.

DAI often occurs after TBI and is characterized by loss of consciousness and extensive axonal damage in the cerebral hemispheres, cerebellum, and brain stem. White matter axons are particularly susceptible to injury following TBI. The shear stress caused by head trauma on white matter axons can result in their rupture, leading to disrupted transport and subsequent physiological changes such as swelling. Almost all patients with severe TBI present with DAI [93]. Studies have demonstrated that axonal abnormalities persist in the brains of TBI patients for years after the initial injury, and DAI may trigger long-term progressive neurodegenerative processes [94].

4.2.3 Posttraumatic epilepsy (PTE)

Posttraumatic epilepsy (PTE) is a common symptom following traumatic brain injury (TBI), with approximately 30% of severe TBI patients developing PTE [95]. About 80% of PTE patients experience seizures within 2 years after the initial injury [96]. Risk factors for PTE include the severity of brain injury, acute cerebral or subdural hematoma, diffuse hydrocephalus, and penetrating brain injury [97]. Posttraumatic seizures (PTS) occur once after head trauma, while PTE is characterized by recurrent epileptiform symptoms in temporal or frontal lobes that can worsen memory and cognitive impairment, sleep disorders, and depression caused by TBI. Antiepileptic drugs such as phenytoin, phenobarbital, levetiracetam, and carbamazepine are commonly used to prevent acute attacks after TBI.

The occurrence of PTE may be associated with damage to the blood-brain barrier (BBB) and intracranial hemorrhage caused by TBI. Infiltration of red blood cells and blood components leads to hemolysis and breakdown of hemoglobin, resulting in the accumulation of free iron and iron-rich compounds such as heme. Studies have indicated that metals can trigger seizures [98]. Iron and ferrous ions initiate an inflammatory response that enhances the generation of free radicals and fragmentation of mitochondria. Oxidative stress leads to lipid peroxidation, causing damage to lipids and promoting the development of epilepsy. This theory was supported by evidence showing that a model of epilepsy could be created by injecting $FeCl_3$ into mice [99]. In TBI epilepsy models, Nrf2, a transcription factor involved in ferroptosis, is significantly reduced, which promotes the expression of multiple antioxidant, anti-inflammatory, and neuroprotective proteins [100]. NMDA receptor-mediated glutamate excitotoxicity, formation of reactive oxygen species (ROS), subsequent membrane lipid peroxidation, and neuronal cell death can exacerbate cerebral ischemia in TBI patients. Further depolarization results in a lower seizure threshold, leading to seizures [101].

4.2.4 Posttraumatic hydrocephalus

Posttraumatic epilepsy, which is a specific type of hydrocephalus occurring after TBI, was first identified in children by Dandy in 1914 [102]. It is more commonly observed in the pediatric population [103]. The cause of PTH may be associated with intracranial hemorrhage and the adhesion of inflammatory mediators following TBI, affecting the outflow and absorption of cerebrospinal fluid (CSF) [104, 105]. Additionally, iron excess in the brain might also contribute to its occurrence. A study demonstrated that injecting red blood cells into the cisterna magna of dogs resulted in increased iron levels and hydrocephalus formation [106]. Furthermore, another study revealed significantly elevated levels of iron and ferritin in the CSF of SAH patients.

Patients with ubarachnoid hemorrhage (SAH) after TBI are more likely to develop PTH, with a significantly higher risk than patients with other types of TBI [107]. The elevated ferritin may be attributed to the robust inflammatory response in the subarachnoid space, leading to an influx of inflammatory cells and stimulation of ferritin synthesis by inflammatory cytokines. Animal studies have also demonstrated that hemoglobin injection enhances heme oxygenase (HO) activity, accelerates heme metabolism [108, 109], induces erythrocyte lysis, and results in iron overload in the brain. Iron accumulation can contribute to ventricular dilatation. Deferoxamine (DFO), an iron chelator, can upregulate HO-1 expression and reduce acute hydrocephalus caused by ventricular dilatation following TBI [110]. DFO has a concentration-dependent ability to bind and remove iron from ferritin and eliminate approximately 10–15% of iron from saturated transferrin but not from hemoglobin [110]. Additionally, increased lipid peroxidation leads to vascular changes that can also contribute to hydrocephalus development [111].

5. Agents targeting iron and ferroptosis for TBI treatment

Traumatic brain injury (TBI) can result in neuronal damage and even cell death while frequently causing various neurological dysfunction encompassing motor deficits, cognitive impairment, dementia, as well as psychiatric disorders like anxiety and depression. These studies indicate a correlation between iron overload, lipid peroxidation along with GSH depletion with neurodegeneration, and subsequent neurological impairments post-TBI. Here, we summarized an overview of the current research on the treatment of TBI in cases involving ferroptosis (**Figure 4** and **Table 1**).

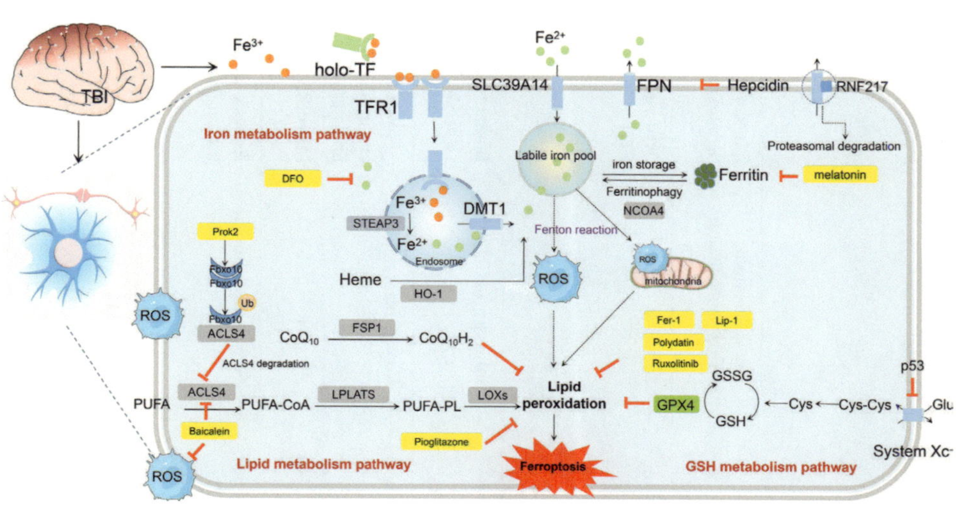

Figure 4.
Scheme of several pathways implicated in ferroptosis in neurons.

Drugs		Targets	Protective effects	Potential mechanisms	References
Deferoxamine (DFO)	Iron chelator	Iron chelator	↓ Brain lesion volume, improve cognitive dysfunction ↑ Cerebral blood flow, improve cerebrovascular function Inhibit ferroptosis and neuroinflammation, Improve neurological dysfunction	↓ FTH, FTL, iron deposition, ROS; ↑ GPx activity	[112–114]
Fer-1	First-generation ferroptosis inhibitor	Inhibitors of lipid peroxidation	↓ Iron deposition, Volume of injury Improve cognitive dysfunction	↓ xCT, FTH, TFR1, FPN, 4HNE, iron deposition, LPO; ↑ GSH	[88, 115, 116]
Melatonin	hormone	Activate MT2 and inhibit FTH	↓ Brain lesion volume, cytoplasmic shrinkage or nuclear pyknosis, neurodegeneration Improve cognitive dysfunction, alleviate anxiety-like behavior	↓ Iron deposition, xCT, COX2, TfR1, Fpn, Nox2, FTH, FTL, 4HNE, MDA, Slc7a11, Ptgs2, ERS; ↑ GSH, MT2; regulate circPtpn14/miR-351-5p/5-LOX signaling	[116, 117]
Baicalein	lipoxygenase inhibitor	Inhibit lipid peroxidation (12/15-LOX inhibitor)	↓ Oxidation of phosphatidylethanolamine, ↑ Neurological function, Improve spatial memory acquisition	↓ Hippocampal neuronal apoptosis, AA/AdA-PE, 15-LOX, ACSL4; ↑ GSH	[118]
Polydatin	lipoxygenase inhibitor	Activate GPX4 pathway and inhibit TFR, inhibit lipid peroxidation	↓ Acute neuronal damage Improve motor deficits and memory dysfunctions	↓ Iron deposition, MDA, Slc7a11, Ptgs2, Atp5g3 ↑ GPX4 activity, Gpx4,	[119]
miR-212-5p	Agonist	Micro-RNA Inhibit Ptgs2	Improve learning and spatial memory	↑ miR-212-5p, Ptgs2; ↓ ferroptosis	[120]
Prokineticin-2 (Prok-2)	Ferroptosis inhibitor	Activate GPX4 pathway Inhibit lipid peroxidation	Inhibits lipid peroxidation to prevent neuronal cell death	↓ biosynthesis of arachidonic acid-phospholipid (a lipid peroxidation substrate, accelerates FBXO10-driven ubiquitination, Ptgs2, ACSL4, ferroptosis ↑ GPX4	[121]
Ruxolitinib	Tyrosine kinase inhibitor	Activate GPX4 pathway and inhibit TfR	↓ Neurodegeneration, brain edema, brain lesion volume, the shrinkage and hyperchromatic morphology; Improve motor deficits and memory dysfunctions, and anxiety-like behaviors	↓ Iron deposition, COX2, TFR1, MDA, 4-HNE↓ ↑ GPX4, GSH, LC3II/I, SCL7A11, FTH	[49]

DOI: http://dx.doi.org/10.5772/intechopen.1005618

Drugs		Targets	Protective effects	Potential mechanisms	References
Anacardic acid	Histone acetyltransferases Inhibitor	Activate GPX4 pathway	Improve neurological function	↓ Ferroptosis	[122]
Orexin-A	G protein-coupled receptor OX1R agonist	Activate Nrf2/HO-1 pathway	↓Brain edema Improve neurological function	↓ Iron overload, ROS; ↑ Nrf2, HO-1, NQO1	[123]
Tetrandrine	Potassium channels activator	Regulate autophagy	Improve neurological function,	↓ MDA, FTH, p62↓; ↑ GSH, GPX4, SCL7A11, BECN1, LC3II/I,	[124]
Hinokitiol	Natural monoterpene small molecule compounds	Activate GPX4	↓ cerebral edema, mNSS, brain contusion lesions; Protect neurons, Improve neurological function	↓ ROS, LPO, Fe^{2+}, MDA, p62; ↑ HO-1, Nrf2, GSH, GPX4, SCL7A11,FTH, BECN1	[125]
Pioglitazone	PPAγ agonist	Activate PPARγ	↓ NSS, injured area, neuronal loss Improve neurological function	↓COX2, DNA; ↑PPARγ	[126]
Netrin-1 (NTN1)	Neurite guidance factors	Activate UNC5B/Nrf2/ GPX4 pathway	Protect neurons, improve neurological function	↓MDA, ROS, ACSL4, LOX ↑Nrf2, GPX4	[127]
Ferristatin II	Iron uptake inhibitors		Protect neurons	↓TfR1, Fe(III), iron overload, MDA, ROS,	[128]
Annexin A5	immune checkpoint inhibitor	Activate NF-kB/ HMGB1andNrf2/ HO-1pathways	Protect neurons, Ameliorates neuroinflammation, oxidative stress and anti-ferroptosis	↓TfR1, Fe(III), iron overload, MDA, ROS, ↑Nrf2, HO-1, SOD activity, ratio of M2/M1,	[129]
N-acetyl serotonin	TrkB agonist	Activate TrkB/PI3K/Akt/ Nrf2 pathway	↓ Iron accumulation in the ipsilateral cortex, Alleviate TBI-induced neurobehavioral deficits, lesion volume and neurodegeneration. Rescue mitochondrial shrinkage, improve neurological function	↓xCT, FTH, TfR1 ↑Nrf2, p-TrkB, p-PI3K, p-AKT, GPX4	[130]
HucMSC-derived exosome	Exosome derived from pluripotent stem cells	Suppress PINK1/Parkin-mediated mitophagy	↓brain edema, neuron death, inhibit neuron apoptosis, pyroptosis and ferroptosis; improve neurological function	↓xCT, FTH, TfR1, MDA, 8-OHdG ↑ Fpn, GPX4	[131]

Table 1.
Agents targeting iron and ferroptosis for TBI treatment.

Given the evidence of iron overload in the brain tissue of TBI patients, drug removal of excessive deposited iron might be an effective therapeutic approach for improving the prognosis of TBI patients. Desferriamine (DFO), as an iron-chelating agent, can bind to excess deposited iron in tissues and cells under pathological conditions. It undergoes oxidative deamination and excreted through the kidney into urine. DFO is commonly employed in clinical treatment for iron overload diseases. Clinical trials have demonstrated that DFO can facilitate hematoma and edema absorption following TBI, while also reducing neuronal degeneration, myelin injury, and inflammation after experimental cerebral hemorrhage. DFO has been shown to alleviate long-term neurotoxicity induced by iron as well as acute cerebral edema caused by TBI in the mouse model, thus alleviating brain damage and cognitive dysfunction in mouse models of TBI [113, 132].

Liproxatin-1 (Lip-1) is a potent antioxidant and ferroptosis inhibitor, comprising amides and sulfonamide subunits that directly inhibit ferroptosis by trapping ROS through the inhibition of xCT or inactivation of GPX4 [94]. It effectively protects cells from ferroptosis. Lip-1 has demonstrated superior efficacy compared to other ferroptosis inhibitors such as DFO and Fer-1. Moreover, Lip-1 exhibits the ability to preserve the integrity of the blood-brain barrier (BBB) in animal models of subarachnoid hemorrhage by inhibiting ferroptosis, suggesting its potential therapeutic value in central nervous system repair by effectively suppressing GPX4-induced oligodendrocyte ferroptosis. In mouse models of TBI, Lip-1 reduces brain injury volume, mitigates neurodegeneration, and improves cognitive dysfunction [116]. These findings provide a promising avenue for clinical treatment of TBI.

Fer-1 is a specific inhibitor of ferroptosis [88, 115, 116], and it has been demonstrated its ability to inhibit cell death in various disease models, including HD, acute brain injury, periabdominal leukomalacia, and kidney failure. It has also shown promising results in stroke and PD models by effectively inhibiting glutamate-induced ferroptosis. In TBI models, intraventricular injection of Fer-1 has been proven to reduce iron accumulation, alleviate neuronal degeneration, and improve cognitive and motor impairment caused by TBI. However, further studies are still needed to validate other clinically applicable methods of administration such as intraperitoneal or intravenous administration.

Melatonin, a hormone secreted by the pineal gland, possesses anti-inflammatory and antioxidant properties. Its lipophilicity enables easy diffusion across cell membranes and subcellular components, effectively blocking a wide range of reactions triggered by TBI, including the ferroptosis pathway. Recent studies have demonstrated that melatonin improves neurological dysfunction following TBI by reducing iron deposition and neurodegeneration [116]. Furthermore, it has been shown that melatonin can effectively enhance nerve function and alleviate motor dysfunction after TBI through inhibition of ferritin heavy chain-mediated ferroptosis [117].

Baicalin (BAI) is a natural flavonoid compound found in the scutellaria plant. It acts as a polyphenol antioxidant and 12/15-LOX inhibitor, possessing anti-inflammatory and antioxidant effects that are widely utilized in clinical practice. Numerous studies have demonstrated the diverse physiological and pharmacological effects of BAI. BAI has been shown to be effective in treating cerebral ischemia by reducing cerebral infarction size and improving neurological deficits in rats with focal cerebral ischemia. Furthermore, it significantly enhances motor function scores and improves motor coordination in animal models after cerebral ischemia, potentially through its involvement in regulating synaptic plasticity and axon growth. Additionally, when injected into the brain tissue of TBI mice, BAI improves memory dysfunction following TBI [120].

Polydatin is a plant extract known for its potent antioxidant and neuroprotective effects. Studies conducted on mouse models of traumatic brain injury (TBI) have demonstrated that polydatin can safeguard neurons, enhance motor deficits in these models, reverse the accumulation of free iron, increase MDA levels, and reduce GPX4 activity in affected brain regions. In vitro studies have also revealed that polydatin can effectively counteract the damage caused by chlormethemoglobin-induced oxidative stress on Neuro2A cells [118].

miR-212-5p, found in various tissues, plays a crucial role in synaptic plasticity, memory formation, and maintaining the integrity of the blood-brain barrier in the brain. In HT-22 and neuro2A cell lines, overexpression of miR-212-5p has been shown to mitigate iron-induced ferroptosis, while downregulation of miR-212-5p promotes ferroptosis through targeting prostaglandin intracperoxidase synthase 2 (PTGS2) [119]. Furthermore, it has been demonstrated that miR-212-5p can significantly enhance spatial learning and memory abilities in TBI mice [119], suggesting its potential to alleviate neuronal iron-induced ferroptosis by targeting PTGS2.

Prokineticin-2 (Prok2) is an important secreted protein likely involved in the pathogenesis of several acute and chronic neurological diseases through currently unidentified regulatory mechanisms. Following traumatic brain injury, neurons undergo mechanical damage which triggers multiple secondary responses including cell death programs such as ferroptosis. It was reported that Prok2 prevents neuronal cell death by inhibiting the biosynthesis of lipid peroxidation substrates, arachidonic acid-phospholipids, via accelerated F-box only protein 10 (Fbxo10)-driven ubiquitination and degradation of long-chain-fatty-acid-CoA ligase 4 (Acsl4), thereby suppressing lipid peroxidation. Mice injected with adeno-associated virus-Prok2 before controlled cortical impact injury exhibit reduced neuronal degeneration and improved motor and cognitive functions [121].

Ruxolitinib, a JAK1/2 inhibitor, is utilized for treating myeloid fibroma. Research has demonstrated that rusotinib exerts neuroprotective effects by inhibiting the JAK-STAT pathway in experimental TBI models [49]. Additionally, it can reduce iron deposition, neurodegeneration, brain edema, and brain injury volume in TBI model mice. This is evidenced by improved motor deficits, memory dysfunction, and anxiety-like behaviors.

Sumac acid (AA), the natural component extracted from cashew nut shells, has been found to have neuroprotective effects in cases of traumatic brain injury. Studies conducted on mouse models with TBI have shown that AA has a strong inhibitory effect on ferroptosis, significantly reducing neural function damage and cognitive impairment caused by TBI [122].

Orexin A (OXA) has been shown to have a protective effect against neuronal damage in various neurological diseases. Studies indicate that OXA effectively inhibits brain tissue injury and nerve function deficits in rats with traumatic brain injury (TBI), while also reducing oxidative stress and iron deposition in the cerebral cortex of these rats. Additionally, OXA may reduce brain damage after TBI by activating the Nrf2/HO-1 signaling pathway, which helps prevent iron-induced ferroptosis [123].

Tetrandrine (Tet) is a natural bibenzyl isoquinoline alkaloid that exhibits promising anticancer, anti-inflammatory, and analgesic properties [124]. Tet effectively mitigates neurotoxicity in 5XFAD mice with cognitive dysfunction by suppressing microglial inflammatory activation. Furthermore, it can alleviate subacute neuronal damage caused by ischemia/reperfusion (I/R-) through the reduction of oxidative stress, apoptosis, and autophagy. Additionally, Tet treatment improves modified NSS (mNSS) scores following traumatic brain injury (TBI), thereby alleviating cerebral contusions and edema in TBI mice [124]. Tet has the potential to ameliorate TBI by attenuating iron-induced cell death via autophagy activation. These findings suggest that Tet may hold promise as a clinical drug for treating TBI.

Hinokitiol (β-thujaplicin, HIK) is a natural monoterpene small molecule that possesses various biological effects, including antibacterial, anti-inflammatory, and anti-tumor activities. Studies have demonstrated that cypress oleophenol can mitigate glutamate-induced intracellular reactive oxygen species (ROS), lipid peroxidation, and Fe^{2+} accumulation in HT-22 cells. Furthermore, it upregulates the expression of heme oxygenase-1 (HO-1), promotes the nuclear translocation of nuclear factor erythroid 2-related factor 2 (Nrf2), inhibits microglia and astrocyte activation after traumatic brain injury (TBI). Additionally, cypress oleophenol significantly reduces brain tissue damage and neuronal loss while alleviating iron deposition in an in vivo TBI model constructed by controlled cortical impact (CCI), thereby mitigating nerve damage. These findings suggest that cypress oleophenol exhibits neuroprotective effects by rescuing cells from TBI-induced neuronal iron enrichment. Moreover, Hyacinol effectively reduces neuronal damage through activation of the Nrf2/Keap1/HO-1 signaling pathway, highlighting its potential as a therapeutic candidate for TBI [125].

Pioglitazone is a specific agonist for peroxisome proliferator-activated receptor-γ (PPARγ), which has been shown to have a protective effect against damage in the central nervous system [126]. PPARγ levels are reduced in neurons that have undergone iron-induced cell death after traumatic brain injury (TBI), but pioglitazone can reverse this reduction [126]. Further studies have demonstrated that PPARγ activation can prevent iron-induced neuronal death. Administration of pioglitazone effectively reduces oxidative damage, as well as nerve severity scores (NSS), damaged areas, and neuronal loss in TBI mice. These findings suggest that pioglitazone may have potential therapeutic effects against iron-induced cell death in the treatment of TBI. Additionally, rosiglitazone (RSG), another PPARγ agonist, exhibits similar neuroprotective effects to pioglitazone by reducing inflammation and neuronal loss after TBI, inhibiting autophagy and apoptosis in cortical neurons. This suggests that RSG could also be used to improve clinical treatment outcomes for TBI patients.

Mouse models demonstrated an upregulation of Netrin-1 (NTN1) mRNA and protein levels following TBI. The administration of NTN1 shRNA resulted in an increase in the number of FJB-positive cells, as well as elevated levels of malondialdehyde (MDA) and reactive oxygen species (ROS). Conversely, the application of NTN1 recombinants had the opposite effect. Furthermore, knockdowns or inhibition of GPX4, Nrf2, and UNC5B counteracted the effects caused by NTN1 recombinants. Intravenous administration of NTN1 recombination reduced neuronal loss after CCI and improved motor and cognitive function [127]. Therefore, it can be concluded that NTN1 exhibits a neuroprotective effect after TBI while inhibiting iron enrichment through activation of the UNC5B/Nrf2 pathway. These findings may offer potential treatment strategies for TBI.

Ferristatin II (Fer-II) is a substance that inhibits iron uptake and TfR1, leading to the down-regulation of TfR1 through receptor degradation. When administered, Fer-II can reduce the expression of TfR1 in neurons, which helps protect them from damage and neurodegeneration caused by TBI [98]. The molecular mechanism behind Fer-II involves reducing Fe3+ content and iron deposits; reversing the expression of proteins related to iron homeostasis such as R1 and lipid peroxidation genes; and lowering high levels of MDA after TBI [128].

When recombinant Annexin A5 (A5) was administered via the tail vein in TBI mice, it exhibited ameliorative effects on neurological deficits, weight loss, cerebral hypoperfusion, cerebral edema, blood-brain barrier disruption, neuronal apoptosis, and iron-induced cell death. Moreover, A5 effectively attenuated neuronal iron accumulation, p53-mediated cell death, and oxidative stress damage. Additionally, A5 downregulated the HMGB1 and NF-kB signaling pathways while upregulating the nuclear factor erythroid 2-related factor 2 (Nrf2) and heme oxygenase-1 (HO-1) pathway. Collectively, these findings demonstrate that A5 exerts neuroprotective effects in traumatic brain injury by modulating the NF-kB/HMGB1 pathway and Nrf2/HO-1 antioxidant system to mitigate neuroinflammation, oxidative stress damage, and ferroptosis [129].

The N-acetyl-5-hydroxytryptamine (NAS), acting as a TrkB agonist and direct melatonin precursor, exhibits multiple advantageous effects on traumatic brain injury (TBI) [130]. Administration of NAS reduces TBI-induced neurobehavioral deficits, lesion volume, and neurodegeneration. Moreover, NAS effectively mitigates TBI-induced mitochondrial contraction, alterations in iron enrichment-related molecular expression, and iron accumulation in the ipsilateral cortex. Additionally, NAS activates the TrkB/PI3K/Akt/Nrf2 pathway in mouse models of TBI. Inhibition of PI3K and Nrf2 weakens the protective effect of NAS on iron enrichment both in vitro and in vivo. These findings suggest that the TrkB agonist therapy with NAS improves brain function following TBI by inhibiting iron enrichment through activation of the PI3K/Akt/Nrf2/Fth pathway. Consequently, these results provide evidence supporting the potential use of NAS as a promising agent for combating iron enrichment during further treatment of TBI.

Researchers established mouse and neuronal models of traumatic brain injury (TBI). Following treatment with exosomes derived from human umbilical cord mesenchymal stem cells (HUCMSCs), it was observed that exosome therapy can enhance neural function post-TBI, mitigate brain edema, and alleviate brain damage. Administration of exosomes suppressed TBI-induced cellular death, apoptosis, pyroptosis, and ferroptosis. Mitochondrial autophagy mediated by the PINK1/Parkin pathway plays a pivotal role in neuroprotection following TBI [131].

6. Conclusions and prospects

The excessive accumulation of iron and ferroptosis, along with disturbances in iron metabolism, is closely associated with traumatic brain injury (TBI). Iron overload can lead to cell death through processes like ferroptosis and autophagy. It also contributes to the phosphorylation of tau protein in brain tissue, leading to the formation of neurofibrillary tangles. Furthermore, it increases the risk of neurodegenerative diseases such as Alzheimer's disease and Parkinson's disease among TBI patients. The potential for neural network damage is also a concern. However, our current understanding of these processes in TBI remains in its early stages, underscoring the importance of delving deeper into their intrinsic relationship.

There are many aspects worth considering. Firstly, in terms of translational medicine, the majority of existing studies primarily focus on a singular factor, and the strategies that can be effectively translated into treatments remain immature. What is the specific regulatory mechanism of ferroptosis on the clinical manifestations of TBI? Sole treatment with antioxidants and anti-excitatory amino acids cannot alleviate cell damage induced by iron overload. Correspondingly, there are certain limitations to improving cognitive function. This suggests that comprehensive consideration of multiple factors is more suitable for selecting clinical treatments. Although iron chelators have been utilized in treating diseases related to iron overload, they have not yet been formally employed in clinical treatment for TBI patients. Rigorous clinical experiments are required to verify their efficacy, which constitutes a long-term project necessitating multi-party cooperation. Secondly, regarding mechanism research, most experimental animal models are used to simulate the pathophysiological characteristics of TBI in humans; while some substances with protective effects on nerve function have been discovered, these animal models fail to fully reflect the complete pathological characteristics observed in humans [112]. The role of iron in the production of ROS and neurotoxicity requires further investigation. Iron chelators are currently only utilized experimentally due to their nephrotoxic and cardiotoxic effects. The clinical application and long-term prognosis of iron chelation therapy in TBI patients also deserve further study. Most likely, the investigation of drug research targeting ferroptosis holds the potential to usher in a new era in the treatment of traumatic brain injury.

Acknowledgements

This work was supported by grants from Medicine and Health Science and Technology Plan Projects of Zhejiang Province (YS, 2020PY029, 2023KY1227), Science and Technology Innovation Special Project of Jiaxing Science and Technology Bureau (YS, 2020AY30003), Key Research Projects of the Affiliated Hospital of Zhejiang Chinese Medical University (YS, 2022FSYYZZ22) and Jiaxing Key Laboratory of Diabetic Angiopathy Research; Jiaxing Key Laboratory of Integrative Rehabilitation of Cerebrovascular Disease.

Conflict of interest

The authors declare no conflict of interest.

Author details

Lifeng Qian[1†], Sunfeng Pan[2†], Yanbing Feng[3†], Hanqiang Shi[4], Lie Xiong[5], Fuxiang Zhu[6], Yanbo Shi[7*] and Zhongwei Yu[6*]

1 Jiaxing Key Laboratory of Integrative Rehabilitation of Cerebrovascular Disease, Zhejiang Chinese Medical University Affiliated Jiaxing Traditional Chinese Medicine Hospital, Zhejiang, China

2 Department of Burns and Plastic Surgery, Zhejiang Chinese Medical University Affiliated Jiaxing Traditional Chinese Medicine Hospital, Jiaxing Key Laboratory of Diabetic Angiopathy Research, Jiaxing Burn and Wound Repair Therapy Center, Jiaxing, Zhejiang, China

3 Department of Ophthalmology, Jiaxing Key Laboratory of Diabetic Angiopathy Research, Zhejiang Chinese Medical University Affiliated Jiaxing Traditional Chinese Medicine Hospital, Zhejiang, China

4 Jiaxing Key Laboratory of Diabetic Angiopathy Research, Central Laboratory of Molecular Medicine Center, Jiaxing Traditional Chinese Medicine Hospital, Jiaxing, Zhejiang, China

5 Central Laboratory of Molecular Medicine Center, Jiaxing Traditional Chinese Medicine Hospital, Jiaxing Key Laboratory of Diabetic Angiopathy Research, Jiaxing, Zhejiang, China

6 Jiaxing Key Laboratory of Diabetic Angiopathy Research, Jiaxing, Zhejiang, China

7 Central Laboratory of Molecular Medicine Center, Zhejiang Chinese Medical University Affiliated Jiaxing Traditional Chinese Medicine Hospital, Jiaxing Key Laboratory of Diabetic Angiopathy Research, Jiaxing, Zhejiang, China

*Address all correspondence to: shiyanbocas@163.com and 13515731616@139.com

†These authors are contributed equally.

References

[1] Toklu HZ et al. Oxidative stress, brain edema, blood–brain barrier permeability, and autonomic dysfunction from traumatic brain injury. In: Kobeissy FH, editor. Brain Neurotrauma: Molecular, Neuropsychological, and Rehabilitation Aspects. Boca Raton (FL): CRC Press/ Taylor & Francis; 2015.Chapter 5. PMID: 26269897

[2] Lee S et al. The incremental induction of neuroprotective properties by multiple therapeutic strategies for primary and secondary neural injury. International Journal of Molecular Sciences. 2015;**16**(8):19657-19670

[3] McKee AC et al. The neuropathology of chronic traumatic encephalopathy. Brain Pathology. 2015;**25**(3):350-364

[4] Kanaan NM et al. Characterization of early pathological tau conformations and phosphorylation in chronic traumatic encephalopathy. Journal of Neuropathology and Experimental Neurology. 2016;**75**(1):19-34

[5] Bouras C et al. A laser microprobe mass analysis of brain aluminum and iron in dementia pugilistica: Comparison with Alzheimer's disease. European Neurology. 1997;**38**(1):53-58

[6] Hui Y et al. Long-term overexpression of heme oxygenase 1 promotes tau aggregation in mouse brain by inducing tau phosphorylation. Journal of Alzheimer's Disease. 2011;**26**(2):299-313

[7] Ke Y, Qian ZM. Brain iron metabolism: Neurobiology and neurochemistry. Progress in Neurobiology. 2007;**83**(3):149-173

[8] Ward RJ et al. The role of iron in brain ageing and neurodegenerative disorders. Lancet Neurology. 2014;**13**(10):1045-1060

[9] Dixon SJ et al. Ferroptosis: An iron-dependent form of nonapoptotic cell death. Cell. 2012;**149**(5):1060-1072

[10] Shichiri M. The role of lipid peroxidation in neurological disorders. Journal of Clinical Biochemistry and Nutrition. 2014;**54**(3):151-160

[11] Cand F, Verdetti J. Superoxide dismutase, glutathione peroxidase, catalase, and lipid peroxidation in the major organs of the aging rats. Free Radical Biology & Medicine. 1989;**7**(1):59-63

[12] Khan JY, Black SM. Developmental changes in murine brain antioxidant enzymes. Pediatric Research. 2003;**54**(1):77-82

[13] Dringen R et al. The pivotal role of astrocytes in the metabolism of iron in the brain. Neurochemical Research. 2007;**32**(11):1884-1890

[14] Shoham S, Youdim MB. Iron involvement in neural damage and microgliosis in models of neurodegenerative diseases. Cellular and Molecular Biology (Noisy-le-Grand). 2000;**46**(4):743-760

[15] Salvador GA. Iron in neuronal function and dysfunction. BioFactors. 2010;**36**(2):103-110

[16] Singh N et al. Brain iron homeostasis: From molecular mechanisms to clinical significance and therapeutic opportunities. Antioxidants & Redox Signaling. 2014;**20**(8):1324-1363

[17] Rouault TA, Cooperman S. Brain iron metabolism. Seminars in Pediatric Neurology. 2006;**13**(3):142-148

[18] Malecki EA et al. Existing and emerging mechanisms for transport of iron and manganese to the brain. Journal of Neuroscience Research. 1999;**56**(2):113-122

[19] Connor JR, Menzies SL. Relationship of iron to oligodendrocytes and myelination. Glia. 1996;**17**(2):83-93

[20] Smith KJ, Kapoor R, Felts PA. Demyelination: The role of reactive oxygen and nitrogen species. Brain Pathology. 1999;**9**(1):69-92

[21] Todorich B, Zhang X, Connor JR. H-ferritin is the major source of iron for oligodendrocytes. Glia. 2011;**59**(6):927-935

[22] Lane DJ et al. Two routes of iron accumulation in astrocytes: Ascorbate-dependent ferrous iron uptake via the divalent metal transporter (DMT1) plus an independent route for ferric iron. The Biochemical Journal. 2010;**432**(1):123-132

[23] Todorich B et al. Tim-2 is the receptor for H-ferritin on oligodendrocytes. Journal of Neurochemistry. 2008;**107**(6):1495-1505

[24] McKie AT et al. A novel duodenal iron-regulated transporter, IREG1, implicated in the basolateral transfer of iron to the circulation. Molecular Cell. 2000;**5**(2):299-309

[25] Fillebeen C et al. Tumor necrosis factor-alpha increases lactoferrin transcytosis through the blood-brain barrier. Journal of Neurochemistry. 1999;**73**(6):2491-2500

[26] Moroo I et al. Identification of a novel route of iron transcytosis across the mammalian blood-brain barrier. Microcirculation. 2003;**10**(6):457-462

[27] Klomp LW et al. Ceruloplasmin gene expression in the murine central nervous system. The Journal of Clinical Investigation. 1996;**98**(1):207-215

[28] Attieh ZK et al. Ceruloplasmin ferroxidase activity stimulates cellular iron uptake by a trivalent cation-specific transport mechanism. The Journal of Biological Chemistry. 1999;**274**(2):1116-1123

[29] Richardson DR. Role of ceruloplasmin and ascorbate in cellular iron release. The Journal of Laboratory and Clinical Medicine. 1999;**134**(5):454-465

[30] Carlson ES et al. Perinatal iron deficiency results in altered developmental expression of genes mediating energy metabolism and neuronal morphogenesis in hippocampus. Hippocampus. 2007;**17**(8):679-691

[31] Wang Y, Wu Y, Li T, Wang X, Zhu C. Iron metabolism and brain development in premature infants. Frontiers in Physiology. 25 Apr 2019;**10**:463. DOI: 10.3389/fphys.2019.00463. PMID: 31105583; PMCID: PMC6494966

[32] Harris ZL et al. Aceruloplasminemia: Molecular characterization of this disorder of iron metabolism. Proceedings of the National Academy of Sciences of the United States of America. 1995;**92**(7):2539-2543

[33] Andrews NC. Disorders of iron metabolism. The New England Journal of Medicine. 1999;**341**(26):1986-1995

[34] Daglas M, Adlard PA. The involvement of iron in traumatic brain injury and neurodegenerative disease. Frontiers in Neuroscience. 2018;**12**:981

[35] Fang X et al. Loss of cardiac ferritin H facilitates cardiomyopathy via

Slc7a11-mediated Ferroptosis. Circulation Research. 2020;**127**(4):486-501

[36] Kagan VE et al. Oxidized arachidonic and adrenic PEs navigate cells to ferroptosis. Nature Chemical Biology. 2017;**13**(1):81-90

[37] Yang WS et al. Regulation of ferroptotic cancer cell death by GPX4. Cell. 2014;**156**(1-2):317-331

[38] Doll S et al. FSP1 is a glutathione-independent ferroptosis suppressor. Nature. 2019;**575**(7784):693-698

[39] Bersuker K et al. The CoQ oxidoreductase FSP1 acts parallel to GPX4 to inhibit ferroptosis. Nature. 2019;**575**(7784):688-692

[40] Kraft VAN et al. GTP cyclohydrolase 1/tetrahydrobiopterin counteract ferroptosis through lipid remodeling. ACS Central Science. 2020;**6**(1):41-53

[41] Soula M et al. Metabolic determinants of cancer cell sensitivity to canonical ferroptosis inducers. Nature Chemical Biology. 2020;**16**(12):1351-1360

[42] Mao C et al. DHODH-mediated ferroptosis defence is a targetable vulnerability in cancer. Nature. 2021;**593**(7860):586-590

[43] Bai Y et al. Lipid storage and lipophagy regulates ferroptosis. Biochemical and Biophysical Research Communications. 2019;**508**(4):997-1003

[44] Doll S et al. ACSL4 dictates ferroptosis sensitivity by shaping cellular lipid composition. Nature Chemical Biology. 2017;**13**(1):91-98

[45] Wenzel SE et al. PEBP1 wardens ferroptosis by enabling lipoxygenase generation of lipid death signals. Cell. 2017;**171**(3):628-641 e26

[46] Bacon BR et al. The pathology of hepatic iron overload: A free radical–mediated process? Hepatology. 1990;**11**(1):127-137

[47] Wang H et al. Characterization of ferroptosis in murine models of hemochromatosis. Hepatology. 2017;**66**(2):449-465

[48] Yu Y et al. Hepatic transferrin plays a role in systemic iron homeostasis and liver ferroptosis. Blood. 2020;**136**(6):726-739

[49] Chen X et al. Ruxolitinib exerts neuroprotection via repressing ferroptosis in a mouse model of traumatic brain injury. Experimental Neurology. 2021;**342**:113762

[50] Feng H et al. Transferrin receptor is a specific Ferroptosis marker. Cell Reports. 2020;**30**(10):3411-3423 e7

[51] Bao WD et al. Loss of ferroportin induces memory impairment by promoting ferroptosis in Alzheimer's disease. Cell Death and Differentiation. 2021;**28**(5):1548-1562

[52] Bao WD et al. Targeting miR-124/ferroportin signaling ameliorated neuronal cell death through inhibiting apoptosis and ferroptosis in aged intracerebral hemorrhage murine model. Aging Cell. 2020;**19**(11):e13235

[53] Protchenko O et al. Iron chaperone poly rC binding protein 1 protects mouse liver from lipid peroxidation and steatosis. Hepatology. 2021;**73**(3):1176-1193

[54] Hou W et al. Autophagy promotes ferroptosis by degradation of ferritin. Autophagy. 2016;**12**(8):1425-1428

[55] Gao M et al. Ferroptosis is an autophagic cell death process. Cell Research. 2016;**26**(9):1021-1032

[56] Ray SK et al. Molecular mechanisms in the pathogenesis of traumatic brain injury. Histology and Histopathology. 2002;**17**(4):1137-1152

[57] Johnson VE et al. Axonal pathology in traumatic brain injury. Experimental Neurology. 2013;**246**:35-43

[58] Stocchetti N et al. Severe traumatic brain injury: Targeted management in the intensive care unit. Lancet Neurology. 2017;**16**(6):452-464

[59] Andersen HH et al. Iron deposits in the chronically inflamed central nervous system and contributes to neurodegeneration. Cellular and Molecular Life Sciences. 2014;**71**(9):1607-1622

[60] Nunez MT et al. Iron toxicity in neurodegeneration. Biometals. 2012;**25**(4):761-776

[61] Thirupathi A et al. Brain iron metabolism and CNS diseases. Advances in Experimental Medicine and Biology. 2019;**1173**:1-19

[62] Dheen ST et al. Microglial activation and its implications in the brain diseases. Current Medicinal Chemistry. 2007;**14**(11):1189-1197

[63] Sulhan S et al. Neuroinflammation and blood–brain barrier disruption following traumatic brain injury: Pathophysiology and potential therapeutic targets. Journal of Neuroscience Research. 2020;**98**(1):19-28

[64] Chodobski A et al. Blood-brain barrier pathophysiology in traumatic brain injury. Translational Stroke Research. 2011;**2**(4):492-516

[65] Price L et al. Blood–brain barrier pathophysiology following traumatic brain injury. In: Laskowitz D, Grant G, editors. Translational Research in Traumatic Brain Injury. Boca Raton (FL): CRC Press/Taylor and Francis Group; 2016. Chapter 4. PMID: 26583184

[66] Lieblein-Boff JC et al. Neonatal *E. Coli* infection causes neuro-behavioral deficits associated with hypomyelination and neuronal sequestration of iron. The Journal of Neuroscience. 2013;**33**(41):16334-16345

[67] Raha-Chowdhury R et al. Expression and cellular localization of hepcidin mRNA and protein in normal rat brain. BMC Neuroscience. 2015;**16**:24

[68] Fischer TD et al. Altered mitochondrial dynamics and TBI pathophysiology. Frontiers in Systems Neuroscience. 2016;**10**:29

[69] Wilde EA et al. Diffusion tensor imaging of the cingulum bundle in children after traumatic brain injury. Developmental Neuropsychology. 2010;**35**(3):333-351

[70] Palmer AM et al. Traumatic brain injury-induced excitotoxicity assessed in a controlled cortical impact model. Journal of Neurochemistry. 1993;**61**(6):2015-2024

[71] Osteen CL et al. Injury-induced alterations in N-methyl-D-aspartate receptor subunit composition contribute to prolonged 45calcium accumulation following lateral fluid percussion. Neuroscience. 2004;**128**(2):305-322

[72] Abdalkader M et al. Targeting Nrf2 to suppress ferroptosis and mitochondrial dysfunction in neurodegeneration. Frontiers in Neuroscience. 2018;**12**:466

[73] Jha RM et al. Pathophysiology and treatment of cerebral edema in traumatic brain injury. Neuropharmacology. 2019;**145**(Pt B):230-246

[74] Winkler EA et al. Cerebral edema in traumatic brain injury: Pathophysiology and prospective therapeutic targets. Neurosurgery Clinics of North America. 2016;**27**(4):473-488

[75] Marmarou A. Pathophysiology of traumatic brain edema: Current concepts. Acta Neurochirurgica. Supplement. 2003;**86**:7-10

[76] Simard JM et al. Brain oedema in focal ischaemia: Molecular pathophysiology and theoretical implications. Lancet Neurology. 2007;**6**(3):258-268

[77] Unterberg AW et al. Edema and brain trauma. Neuroscience. 2004;**129**(4):1021-1029

[78] Zhang Z et al. Glutathione peroxidase 4 participates in secondary brain injury through mediating ferroptosis in a rat model of intracerebral hemorrhage. Brain Research. 2018;**1701**:112-125

[79] Hall ED et al. Antioxidant therapies for traumatic brain injury. Neurotherapeutics. 2010;**7**(1):51-61

[80] Chan PH et al. Induction of brain edema following intracerebral injection of arachidonic acid. Annals of Neurology. 1983;**13**(6):625-632

[81] Millis SR et al. Long-term neuropsychological outcome after traumatic brain injury. The Journal of Head Trauma Rehabilitation. 2001;**16**(4):343-355

[82] Lange RT et al. Post-traumatic stress disorder is associated with neuropsychological outcome but not white matter integrity after mild traumatic brain injury. Journal of Neurotrauma. 2021;**38**(1):63-73

[83] Dougan BK et al. Athletes' age, sex, and years of education moderate the acute neuropsychological impact of sports-related concussion: A meta-analysis. Journal of the International Neuropsychological Society. 2014;**20**(1):64-80

[84] Vincent AS et al. Cognitive changes and dementia risk after traumatic brain injury: Implications for aging military personnel. Alzheimers Dement. 2014;**10**(3 Suppl):S174-S187

[85] Gupta PK et al. Subtypes of post-traumatic epilepsy: Clinical, electrophysiological, and imaging features. Journal of Neurotrauma. 2014;**31**(16):1439-1443

[86] Ansari MA et al. Oxidative stress and modification of synaptic proteins in hippocampus after traumatic brain injury. Free Radical Biology & Medicine. 2008;**45**(4):443-452

[87] Maher P. Potentiation of glutathione loss and nerve cell death by the transition metals iron and copper: Implications for age-related neurodegenerative diseases. Free Radical Biology & Medicine. 2018;**115**:92-104

[88] Xie BS et al. Inhibition of ferroptosis attenuates tissue damage and improves long-term outcomes after traumatic brain injury in mice. CNS Neuroscience & Therapeutics. 2019;**25**(4):465-475

[89] Fleminger S et al. Head injury as a risk factor for Alzheimer's disease: The evidence 10 years on; a partial replication. Journal of Neurology, Neurosurgery, and Psychiatry. 2003;**74**(7):857-862

[90] Gomez-Isla T et al. Neuronal loss correlates with but exceeds neurofibrillary tangles in Alzheimer's disease. Annals of Neurology. 1997;**41**(1):17-24

[91] Yao P et al. Hippocampal neuronal ferroptosis involved in cognitive dysfunction in rats with sepsis-related encephalopathy through the Nrf2/GPX4 signaling pathway. Zhonghua Wei Zhong Bing Ji Jiu Yi Xue. 2019;**31**(11):1389-1394

[92] Zlokovic BV. Neurovascular pathways to neurodegeneration in Alzheimer's disease and other disorders. Nature Reviews Neuroscience. 2011;**12**(12):723-738

[93] Povlishock JT et al. Update of neuropathology and neurological recovery after traumatic brain injury. The Journal of Head Trauma Rehabilitation. 2005;**20**(1):76-94

[94] Chen XH et al. A lack of amyloid beta plaques despite persistent accumulation of amyloid beta in axons of long-term survivors of traumatic brain injury. Brain Pathology. 2009;**19**(2):214-223

[95] Bao YH et al. Post-traumatic seizures exacerbate histopathological damage after fluid-percussion brain injury. Journal of Neurotrauma. 2011;**28**(1):35-42

[96] Verellen RM et al. Post-traumatic epilepsy: An overview. Therapy. 2010;7(5):527-531

[97] Curia G et al. Modeling post-traumatic epilepsy for therapy development. In: Laskowitz D, Grant G, editors. Translational Research in Traumatic Brain Injury. Boca Raton (FL): CRC Press/Taylor and Francis Group; 2016. Chapter 10. PMID: 26583185

[98] Kellner CP et al. The stereotactic intracerebral Hemorrhage underwater blood aspiration (SCUBA) technique for minimally invasive endoscopic intracerebral hemorrhage evacuation. Journal of Neurointerventional Surgery. 2018;**10**(8):771-776

[99] Jyoti A et al. Curcumin protects against electrobehavioral progression of seizures in the iron-induced experimental model of epileptogenesis. Epilepsy & Behavior. 2009;**14**(2):300-308

[100] Ghadiri T et al. Neuronal injury and death following focal mild brain injury: The role of network excitability and seizure. Iranian Journal of Basic Medical Sciences. 2020;**23**(1):63-70

[101] Willmore LJ et al. Posttraumatic epilepsy: Hemorrhage, free radicals and the molecular regulation of glutamate. Neurochemical Research. 2009;**34**(4):688-697

[102] De SN. A study of the changes in the brain in experimental internal hydrocephalus. The Journal of Pathology and Bacteriology. 1950;**62**(2):197-208

[103] Fattahian R et al. Development of posttraumatic hydrocephalus requiring ventriculoperitoneal shunt after decompressive craniectomy for traumatic brain injury: A systematic review and meta-analysis of retrospective studies. Medical Archives. 2018;**72**(3):214-219

[104] Miki T et al. Cause of post-traumatic hydrocephalus because of traumatic aqueduct obstruction in two cases. The Journal of Trauma. 2006;**61**(4):985-989

[105] Shah AH et al. Pathophysiology of acute hydrocephalus after subarachnoid hemorrhage. World Neurosurgery. Sep-Oct 2013;**80**(3-4):304-306. DOI: 10.1016/j.wneu.2013.01.110. Epub 2013 Feb 1. PMID: 23376378

[106] Iwanowski L et al. The effects of subarachnoid injections of iron-containing substances on the central nervous system. Journal of Neuropathology and Experimental Neurology. 1960;**19**:433-448

[107] Chen KH et al. Incidence of hydrocephalus in traumatic brain injury: A nationwide population-based cohort study. Medicine (Baltimore). 2019;**98**(42):e17568

[108] Matz P et al. Heme-oxygenase-1 induction in glia throughout rat brain following experimental subarachnoid hemorrhage. Brain Research. 1996;**713**(1-2):211-222

[109] Turner CP et al. Heme oxygenase-1 is induced in glia throughout brain by subarachnoid hemoglobin. Journal of Cerebral Blood Flow and Metabolism. 1998;**18**(3):257-273

[110] Zhao J et al. Deferoxamine attenuates acute hydrocephalus after traumatic brain injury in rats. Translational Stroke Research. 2014;**5**(5):586-594

[111] Caner H et al. Lipid peroxide level increase in experimental hydrocephalus. Acta Neurochirurgica (Wien). 1993;**121**(1-2):68-71

[112] DeWitt DS et al. Pre-clinical testing of therapies for traumatic brain injury. Journal of Neurotrauma. 2018;**35**(23):2737-2754

[113] Jia H et al. Deferoxamine ameliorates neurological dysfunction by inhibiting ferroptosis and neuroinflammation after traumatic brain injury. Brain Research. 2023;**1812**:148383

[114] Liang Y et al. Deferoxamine reduces endothelial ferroptosis and protects cerebrovascular function after experimental traumatic brain injury. Brain Research Bulletin. 2024;**207**:110878

[115] Fang J et al. Ferroptosis in brain microvascular endothelial cells mediates blood-brain barrier disruption after traumatic brain injury. Biochemical and Biophysical Research Communications. 2022;**619**:34-41

[116] Rui T et al. Deletion of ferritin H in neurons counteracts the protective effect of melatonin against traumatic brain injury-induced ferroptosis. Journal of Pineal Research. 2021;**70**(2):e12704

[117] Wu C et al. A novel mechanism linking ferroptosis and endoplasmic reticulum stress via the circPtpn14/miR-351-5p/5-LOX signaling in melatonin-mediated treatment of traumatic brain injury. Free Radical Biology and Medicine. 2022;**178**:271-294

[118] Huang L et al. Polydatin alleviates traumatic brain injury: Role of inhibiting ferroptosis. Biochemical and Biophysical Research Communications. 2021;**556**:149-155

[119] Xiao X et al. miR-212-5p attenuates ferroptotic neuronal death after traumatic brain injury by targeting Ptgs2. Molecular Brain. 18 Sep 2019;**12**(1):78. DOI: 10.1186/s13041-019-0501-0. PMID: 31533781; PMCID: PMC6749650

[120] Li M et al. Baicalein ameliorates cerebral ischemia-reperfusion injury by inhibiting ferroptosis via regulating GPX4/ACSL4/ACSL3 axis. Chemico-Biological Interactions. 1 Oct 2022;**366**:110137. DOI: 10.1016/j.cbi.2022.110137. Epub 2022 August 31. PMID: 36055377

[121] Bao Z et al. Prokineticin-2 prevents neuronal cell deaths in a model of traumatic brain injury. Nature Communications. 2021;**12**(1):4220

[122] Liu Y et al. Anacardic acid improves neurological deficits in traumatic brain injury by anti-ferroptosis and anti-inflammation. Experimental Neurology. 2023;**370**:114568

[123] Kang J et al. Orexin-A alleviates ferroptosis by activating the Nrf2/HO-1 signaling pathway in traumatic brain injury. Aging (Albany NY). 2024;**16**(4):3404-3419

[124] Liu H et al. Tetrandrine ameliorates traumatic brain injury by regulating autophagy to reduce ferroptosis. Neurochemical Research. 2022;**47**(6):1574-1587

[125] Tang H et al. Protective effects of hinokitiol on neuronal ferroptosis by activating the Keap1/Nrf2/HO-1 pathway in traumatic brain injury. Journal of Neurotrauma. 2024;**41**(5-6):734-750

[126] Liang H et al. Peroxisome proliferator-activated receptor-gamma ameliorates neuronal ferroptosis after traumatic brain injury in mice by inhibiting cyclooxygenase-2. Experimental Neurology. 2022;**354**:114100

[127] Zhang Y et al. Netrin-1 upregulates GPX4 and prevents ferroptosis after traumatic brain injury via the UNC5B/Nrf2 signaling pathway. CNS Neuroscience & Therapeutics. 2023;**29**(1):216-227

[128] Cheng Y et al. Ferristatin II, an iron uptake inhibitor, exerts neuroprotection against traumatic brain injury via suppressing ferroptosis. ACS Chemical Neuroscience. 2022;**13**(5):664-675

[129] Gao Y et al. Annexin A5 ameliorates traumatic brain injury-induced neuroinflammation and neuronal ferroptosis by modulating the NF-kB/HMGB1 and Nrf2/HO-1 pathways. International Immunopharmacology. 2023;**114**:109619

[130] Cheng Y et al. TrkB agonist N-acetyl serotonin promotes functional recovery after traumatic brain injury by suppressing ferroptosis via the PI3K/Akt/Nrf2/Ferritin H pathway. Free Radical Biology and Medicine. 2023;**194**:184-198

[131] Zhang L et al. Human umbilical cord mesenchymal stem cell-derived exosome suppresses programmed cell death in traumatic brain injury via PINK1/Parkin-mediated mitophagy. CNS Neuroscience & Therapeutics. 2023;**29**(8):2236-2258

[132] Zhang L et al. Deferoxamine attenuates iron-induced long-term neurotoxicity in rats with traumatic brain injury. Neurological Sciences. 2013;**34**(5):639-645

Chapter 7

The Research Progress of Molecular Hydrogen in the Treatment of Traumatic Brain Injury: A Review

Jiayuan Zhai and Wanchao Yang

Abstract

Molecular hydrogen, a medical gas with potent antioxidant and anti-inflammatory effects, exhibits significant therapeutic potential for various diseases. Traumatic brain injury (TBI) is often accompanied by extensive cognitive dysfunction, characterized by complex pathogenesis and poor prognosis. Recent studies have demonstrated that inhalation of a high concentration of molecular hydrogen can improve the prognosis of TBI; however, the specific mechanism remains unclear. This article provides a comprehensive review on the mechanisms underlying the action of a high concentration of molecular hydrogen in TBI and discusses its association with AMPK, HDAC5, acetyl-CoA, microglial histone acetylation, and GSK3β/PTEN/Akt axis. These findings offer a theoretical foundation for further experimental and clinical research of molecular hydrogen in TBI treatment.

Keywords: molecular hydrogen, traumatic brain injury, neuroinflammation, microglial histone acetylation, AMPK

1. Introduction

Traumatic brain injury (TBI), also known as cranial injury, is a form of brain tissue damage resulting from trauma that can have significant and far-reaching consequences [1]. It has emerged as a prominent concern in contemporary society. According to statistics, the global annual incidence of moderate to severe traumatic brain injuries leading to disability reaches up to 80,000 individuals [2]. This condition primarily affects children and young adults, making it one of the leading causes of mortality and disability rates in China [2, 3]. Post-traumatic TBI patients often experience a wide range of cognitive dysfunctions including reduced attention span, impaired reasoning abilities, diminished memory capabilities, decreased intellectual functioning, and compromised motor skills. For an extended period, cognitive impairment has been identified as the primary factor contributing toward psychological distress, lifestyle challenges, and societal burdens faced by individuals affected by TBIs [4, 5]. Currently, no effective treatment for cognitive dysfunction in TBIs exists [4, 6, 7]. Therefore, it remains imperative to explore novel therapeutic approaches. In a 2007 publication, Ohsawa reported that the inhalation of 2% molecular hydrogen selectively eliminates hydroxyl (·OH) and peroxynitrite anions, thereby significantly ameliorating oxidative stress injury induced by cerebral ischemia/reperfusion [8]. Subsequently, the medical significance of molecular hydrogen has garnered considerable attention. Moreover, molecular hydrogen possesses attributes such as facile preparation, low cost, rapid onset of action, non-toxicity, and absence of residue, thus, offering promising prospects for its clinical application in the treatment of brain injury disorders. This review mainly introduced the latest research progress in the treatment and underlying mechanisms of molecular hydrogen in TBI to provide new ideas for further experimental and clinical research of molecular hydrogen in TBI treatment.

2. Immune response and regulation following TBI

TBI involves two main pathological stages: primary and secondary brain injury. Primary brain injury results from direct mechanical force during trauma, which damages blood vessels, neurons, and glial cells around the brain tissue, leading to multiple chronic injuries. Over time, these factors trigger secondary brain injury by causing hypoxia and ischemia in the brain tissue resulting in edema of brain cells, increased intracranial pressure, decreased cerebral perfusion pressure further aggravating hypoxia and ischemia. The process of TBI involves various mechanisms such as depolarization and ion homeostasis disorder, neurotransmitter release, mitochondrial dysfunction, nerve cell apoptosis, inflammatory factor release, initiation of immune response among others [9, 10].

Studies have demonstrated that excessive immune regulation following traumatic brain injury often gives rise to a cascade of post-traumatic complications, which constitutes a significant etiology of mortality in TBI patients [11–13]. Microglia, the principal cellular component of the innate immune system within the central nervous system, serves as the first line of defense against injury or disease and plays a pivotal role in neuroinflammation after TBI. Research has indicated that microglial activation within the central nervous system is heterogeneous and contingent upon phenotypic activation, thus capable of exerting cytotoxic or neuroprotective effects [14]. Activated microglia exhibit classical (M1) and alternative (M2) activation phenotypes. M1 microglia demonstrate pro-inflammatory properties through the release of inflammatory mediators associated with cell death. Conversely, M2 phenotype assumes a reparative and protective function by releasing neurotrophic factors and other anti-inflammatory agents. Within an appropriate temporal window, phenotypic conversion from M1/M2 microglia at specific stages may confer therapeutic benefits [15, 16].

More and more evidence indicate that activated microglia play a crucial role in the inflammatory response following TBI [17]. During the secondary injury phase of TBI, M1-type microglia primarily contribute to the damage, whereas M2-type microglia have a neuroprotective effect [18]. Wen et al. discovered that after TBI, there was a significant increase in the M1 phenotype of microglia, accompanied by a decrease in the M2 phenotype. Activation of PPAR-γ by rosiglitazone promoted microglial polarization toward the M2 phenotype, thereby reducing inflammation, alleviating cortical axonal injury, and improving neurological function. Conversely, GW9662 inhibited microglial polarization toward M2 phenotype and exacerbated inflammation and axonal injury [16].

The immune response is traditionally categorized into the innate immune response and adaptive immune response. Following injury, the innate immune system modulates bodily functions to prevent reinfection, a phenomenon known as innate immune memory [19]. Furthermore, immune stimulation can also alter the pathological characteristics following stroke and exert a significant protective effect against cerebral ischemia [20]. The latest evidence also points to a role of the adaptive immune response in the pathogenesis of Alzheimer's disease (AD) [21].

At the same time, studies have also demonstrated that the intrinsic reprogramming of microglia and astrocytes is implicated in innate immune memory, while the activation of innate immune responses plays a pivotal role in stimulating the adaptive immune system [22]. Innate immune training enables innate immune cells to recall prior inflammatory episodes, serving as a crucial mechanism for bone marrow cell plasticity and facilitating subsequent inflammation modulation. Previous investigations have indicated that brain immunological memory primarily relies on microglia, which occurs in response to environmental stimuli and subsequently alters immune responses [23]. Therefore, exploring the regulatory process of microglial immunological memory holds significant implications for post-traumatic neurological function treatment and recovery.

Epigenetic modification involves the regulation of gene expression levels and is considered to be a fundamental component in the pathogenesis of numerous diseases [24]. The regulation of gene expression, known as epigenetics, plays a critical role in maintaining normal cellular function. Histone acetylation serves as one of the key mechanisms involved in this process, promoting an active form of DNA transcription, while histone deacetylation leads to relative transcriptional silence [25]. The epigenetic modification of microglia is triggered by surrounding immune stimulation, resulting in subsequent alterations in the transcription and functionality of associated genes. It has been confirmed that changes occur in histone acetylation modification during the processes of immune memory and immune tolerance within microglia [26, 27].

The efficacy of HDAC inhibitors in increasing histone H3 acetylation and reducing microglial inflammation induced by TBI has been demonstrated. The acetylation status of chromatin histones is dependent on the activity of two enzymes, namely histone acetyltransferase (HAT) and histone deacetylase (HDAC), which compete for lysine residue acetylation within the histones. Typically, HAT functions to acetylate lysine groups in histones, thereby neutralizing their charge and promoting a more open chromatin structure that is transcriptionally active. Conversely, HDAC acts to deacetylate and inhibit transcription. Any alteration in the balance of chromatin acetylation can lead to changes in gene expression regulation patterns [28].

Acetylated histones exert neuroprotective effects by attenuating inflammation and inhibiting neuronal apoptosis, thereby enhancing neurological function in various neurological disorders such as cerebral ischemia [29], brain injury [30], and spinal cord injury [31]. Moumita et al. [32] discovered that the depletion of histone deacetylases HDAC1 and HDAC2 from adult microglia can effectively reduce amyloid plaques and ameliorate spatial learning and memory deficits. In vitro investigations also have revealed that HDAC inhibitors not only decrease inflammatory markers but also mitigate traumatic brain injury-induced reductions in histone H3 acetylation, while exhibiting a tendency to alleviate neuronal degeneration, thus displaying robust neuroprotective properties [28]. Therefore, modulation of histone acetylation can regulate microglial immune memory and consequently contribute to the progression of traumatic brain injury.

3. Molecular hydrogen

Molecular hydrogen is well known as a novel safe and effective antioxidant and anti-inflammatory agent characterized by its ROS scavengingand anti-inflammation abilities by decreasing the level of hydroxyl radicals (·OH), reducing the expressions of pro-inflammatory cytokines and activating anti-oxidative stress and anti-inflammatory pathways in various diseases such as cardiovascular and cerebrovascular diseases [33], tumor [34] and neurodegenerative diseases [35]. Up to know that no endogenous cells capable of directly producing molecular hydrogen have been identified in the human body [36]. Currently, molecular hydrogen can be administered through various methods including inhalation at high or low concentrations, intravenous injection of hydrogen-rich saline, oral administration [37]. Research conducted by Chen et al. [38] suggests that the neuroprotective effects of molecular hydrogen may be positively correlated with its concentration and dosage. Compared to a low concentration inhalation of molecular hydrogen, a high concentration of molecular hydrogen exhibits superior antioxidant stress response, anti-apoptotic properties, and anti-inflammatory effects due to its high diffusivity, excellent biomembrane permeability and tissue dispersion ability. Therefore, inhaling a high concentration of molecular hydrogen can rapidly reach target organs and exert corresponding therapeutic effects.

Randomized controlled clinical studies have demonstrated the neuroprotective effects and high biosafety of molecular hydrogen inhalation in patients with acute cerebral infarction [39]. Additionally, our research team demonstrated that molecular hydrogen inhalation in a high concentration could promoting neurological functional recovery, reducing postoperative brain edema formation, mitigating pathological damage and neuronal apoptosis in brain tissues after TBI [40–43]. Collectively, these findings suggest that molecular hydrogen exhibits substantial protective effects against acute traumatic brain injury by reducing secondary injury, however, further research is needed to elucidate its specific mechanism.

4. Therapeutic effect of a high concentration of molecular hydrogen in TBI

The therapeutic mechanism of molecular hydrogen in TBI is multifaceted, with early studies primarily focusing on its antioxidant, anti-inflammatory, and anti-apoptotic effects. However, in this paper we highlighted the crucial role of immune memory regulation in TBI induced inflammatory response and the therapeutic effect of molecular hydrogen modulating phenotypic changes of microglia, maintaining a dynamic balance between M1 and M2 microglial cells and exerting anti-inflammatory effects in the pathological state of TBI, which may present a novel therapeutic target for TBI.

Studies have demonstrated that activated microglia play a pivotal role in brain injury through the production of various pro-inflammatory cytokines and release of oxidative products [44]. Researches have found that molecular hydrogen exhibits neuroprotective effects by inhibiting the upregulation of M1 microglia and pro-inflammatory cytokines and promoting microglial M2 polarization, thereby demonstrating its neuroprotective properties [45–48]. Consequently, the therapeutic effect molecular hydrogen in TBI may be associated with the modulation of microglial polarization.

The adenosine monophosphate-activated protein kinase (AMPK) serves as an important regulator of cellular energy homeostasis, orchestrating catabolic processes and suppressing anabolic pathways under metabolic stress conditions [49]. It actively participates in the modulation of enzymes involved in overall cellular and organismal energy equilibrium, as well as glucose and lipid metabolism. AMPK exhibits robust expression within neurons, astrocytes, and microglia, exerting diverse functions in promoting M2 polarization of macrophages/microglia [50]. Research has demonstrated that hydrogen-rich saline can enhance M2 polarization of microglia and counteract complement-mediated synaptic loss by activating AMPK, thereby ameliorating behavioral impairments following neonatal hypoxia-ischemia events [46]. In our unpublished data, we also proved that AMPK expression levels were down-regulated following TBI insult, and molecular hydrogen treatment activated AMPK expression and inhibited HDAC5/GSK3β/AKT signaling along with restored neuronal function.

The cofactor acetyl-CoA (CoA), primarily generated through glucose metabolism, is essential for the activity of acetyltransferase. Acetyl-CoA homeostasis plays a crucial role in regulating histone acetylation, which is closely associated with cell proliferation [25]. Previous studies have demonstrated that AMPK maintains target gene expression by modulating both acetyl-CoA levels and chromatin recruitment of BET proteins (Bromodomain and Extra-Terminal domain) [51]. Moreover, Metformin can enhance the expression of brain-derived neurotrophic factor (BDNF) by activating AMPK-mediated histone acetylation, thereby improving stress-induced depression-like behavior [52]. Recent studies have reported that AMPK can also promote the nucleation of HDAC5 by phosphorylating HDAC5 at Ser259 and Ser498 residues, inhibiting its role as a histone deacetylase [53]. Consequently, the loss of AMPK leads to decreased levels of acetyl-CoA and histone acetylation and molecular hydrogen may regulate microglial histone acetylation by inhibiting HDAC5 and increasing acetyl-CoA.

The GSK3β/PTEN/Akt axis and its signaling pathway are implicated in the pathogenesis of TBI [54]. GSK3β protein is a transcriptional product regulated by HDAC, while PTEN acts as a negative regulator of PI3K/Akt signal transduction. Wang et al. [54] have demonstrated that HDAC inhibitors modulate microglia/macrophage polarization through the GSK3β/PTEN/Akt axis to mitigate white matter damage in TBI. By enhancing the expression of GSK3β, HDAC inhibitors facilitate cytoplasmic PTEN phosphorylation/inactivation, thereby suppressing PI3K/Akt signal transduction and potentially exerting anti-inflammatory and phagocytic effects on microglia. Consequently, it is plausible that HDAC5 may regulate microglial polarization and exacerbate TBI by promoting deacetylation of the GSK3β promoter. Activation of the GSK3β/PTEN/Akt axis might represent a downstream mechanism underlying hydrogen treatment for TBI.

5. Summary

Molecular hydrogen, recently proven as an ideal antioxidant and anti-inflammatory substance, exhibiting anti-inflammatory, antioxidant, and anti-apoptotic properties, exerts protective effects against various oxidative stress and inflammatory injuries. It has demonstrated therapeutic potential for a wide range of diseases without any observed toxic side effects. However, the specific mechanism underlying molecular hydrogen treatment for traumatic brain injury (TBI) remains unclear. From preceding text, we can presume that molecular hydrogen can promote microglial histone acetylation and further regulate microglial polarization toward the M2 phenotype through the GSK3β/PTEN/Akt axis, ultimately exerting therapeutic effects on TBI. This concept reveals the epigenetic regulating mechanism of molecular hydrogen targeting TBI treatment, thus providing a theoretical basis for targeted treatment strategies and basic research regarding molecular hydrogen in TBI treatment.

Author details

Jiayuan Zhai[1] and Wanchao Yang[2]*

1 Department of Anesthesiology, The Second Affiliated Hospital of Harbin Medical University, Harbin Medical University, Harbin, Heilongjiang Province, China

2 Department of Anesthesiology, The Sixth Affiliated Hospital of Harbin Medical University, Harbin Medical University, Harbin, Heilongjiang Province, China

*Address all correspondence to: dachao_1980@126.com

References

[1] Capizzi A, Woo J, Verduzco-Gutierrez M. Traumatic brain injury: An overview of epidemiology, pathophysiology, and medical management. The Medical Clinics of North America. 2020;**104**(2):213-238

[2] Jiang JY et al. Traumatic brain injury in China. Lancet Neurology. 2019;**18**(3):286-295

[3] Gao G et al. Clinical characteristics and outcomes in patients with traumatic brain injury in China: A prospective, multicentre, longitudinal, observational study. The Lancet Neurology. 2020;**19**(8):670-677

[4] Lutkenhoff ES et al. The subcortical basis of outcome and cognitive impairment in TBI: A longitudinal cohort study. Neurology. 2020;**95**(17):e2398-e2408

[5] Elder GA. Update on TBI and cognitive impairment in military veterans. Current Neurology and Neuroscience Reports. 2015;**15**(10):68

[6] Rabinowitz AR, Watanabe TK. Pharmacotherapy for treatment of cognitive and neuropsychiatric symptoms after mTBI. The Journal of Head Trauma Rehabilitation. 2020;**35**(1):76-83

[7] Fyfe I. Predicting treatment response in post-TBI cognitive impairment. Nature Reviews Neurology. 2019;**15**(9):492-493

[8] Ohsawa I et al. Hydrogen acts as a therapeutic antioxidant by selectively reducing cytotoxic oxygen radicals. Nature Medicine. 2007;**13**(6):688-694

[9] Kinoshita K. Traumatic brain injury: Pathophysiology for neurocritical care. Journal of Intensive Care. 2016;**4**:29

[10] Maas AIR et al. Traumatic brain injury: Integrated approaches to improve prevention, clinical care, and research. Lancet Neurology. 2017;**16**(12):987-1048

[11] Netea MG et al. Trained immunity: A program of innate immune memory in health and disease. Science. 2016;**352**(6284):aaf1098

[12] Mitroulis I et al. Modulation of myelopoiesis progenitors is an integral component of trained immunity. Cell. 2018;**172**(1-2):147-161.e12

[13] Wang Z, Chen G. Immune regulation in neurovascular units after traumatic brain injury. Neurobiology of Disease. 2023;**179**:106060

[14] Karve IP, Taylor JM, Crack PJ. The contribution of astrocytes and microglia to traumatic brain injury. British Journal of Pharmacology. 2016;**173**(4):692-702

[15] Witcher KG et al. Traumatic brain injury causes chronic cortical inflammation and neuronal dysfunction mediated by microglia. The Journal of Neuroscience. 2021;**41**(7):1597-1616

[16] Wen L et al. Polarization of microglia to the M2 phenotype in a peroxisome proliferator-activated receptor gamma-dependent manner attenuates axonal injury induced by traumatic brain injury in mice. Journal of Neurotrauma. 2018;**35**(19):2330-2340

[17] Balogh ZJ, Marzi I. Novel concepts related to inflammatory complications in polytrauma. European Journal of Trauma and Emergency Surgery. 2018;**44**(3):299-300

[18] Kumar A et al. Microglial/macrophage polarization dynamics

following traumatic brain injury. Journal of Neurotrauma. 2016;**33**(19):1732-1750

[19] Salvador AFM, Kipnis J. Immune response after central nervous system injury. Seminars in Immunology. 2022;**59**:101629

[20] Iadecola C, Anrather J. The immunology of stroke: From mechanisms to translation. Nature Medicine. 2011;**17**(7):796-808

[21] Chen X, Holtzman DM. Emerging roles of innate and adaptive immunity in Alzheimer's disease. Immunity. 2022;**55**(12):2236-2254

[22] Netea MG et al. Innate immune memory: A paradigm shift in understanding host defense. Nature Immunology. 2015;**16**(7):675-679

[23] Wendeln AC et al. Innate immune memory in the brain shapes neurological disease hallmarks. Nature. 2018;**556**(7701):332-338

[24] Chen Y et al. Epigenetic modification of nucleic acids: From basic studies to medical applications. Chemical Society Reviews. 2017;**46**(10):2844-2872

[25] Shvedunova M, Akhtar A. Modulation of cellular processes by histone and non-histone protein acetylation. Nature Reviews Molecular Cell Biology. 2022;**23**(5):329-349

[26] Rodriguez-Zas SL et al. Disruption of microglia histone acetylation and protein pathways in mice exhibiting inflammation-associated depression-like symptoms. Psychoneuroendocrinology. 2018;**97**:47-58

[27] Maleszewska M et al. Sequential changes in histone modifications shape transcriptional responses underlying microglia polarization by glioma. Glia. 2021;**69**(1):109-123

[28] Zhang B et al. HDAC inhibitor increases histone H3 acetylation and reduces microglia inflammatory response following traumatic brain injury in rats. Brain Research. 2008;**1226**:181-191

[29] Aune SE et al. Histone deacetylases exert class-specific roles in conditioning the brain and heart against acute ischemic injury. Frontiers in Neurology. 2015;**6**:145

[30] Liao Y et al. HDAC3 inhibition ameliorates ischemia/reperfusion-induced brain injury by regulating the microglial cGAS-STING pathway. Theranostics. 2020;**10**(21):9644-9662

[31] Chen S et al. Valproic acid attenuates traumatic spinal cord injury-induced inflammation via STAT1 and NF-κB pathway dependent of HDAC3. Journal of Neuroinflammation. 2018;**15**(1):150

[32] Datta M et al. Histone deacetylases 1 and 2 regulate microglia function during development, homeostasis, and neurodegeneration in a context-dependent manner. Immunity. 2018;**48**(3):514-529.e6

[33] Gao Y et al. Hydrogen gas attenuates myocardial ischemia reperfusion injury independent of postconditioning in rats by attenuating endoplasmic reticulum stress-induced autophagy. Cellular Physiology and Biochemistry. 2017;**43**(4):1503-1514

[34] Hirano SI et al. Molecular hydrogen as a novel antitumor agent: Possible mechanisms underlying gene expression. International Journal of Molecular Sciences. 2021;**22**(16):8724

[35] Iketani M, Ohsawa I. Molecular hydrogen as a neuroprotective agent. Current Neuropharmacology. 2017;**15**(2):324-331

[36] Artamonov MY et al. Molecular hydrogen: From molecular effects to stem cells management and tissue regeneration. Antioxidants (Basel, Switzerland). 2023;**12**(3):636

[37] Wu C et al. Molecular hydrogen: An emerging therapeutic medical gas for brain disorders. Molecular Neurobiology. 2023;**60**(4):1749-1765

[38] Chen X et al. Inhalation of hydrogen of different concentrations ameliorates spinal cord injury in mice by protecting spinal cord neurons from apoptosis, oxidative injury and mitochondrial structure damages. Cellular Physiology and Biochemistry. 2018;**47**(1):176-190

[39] Ono H et al. Hydrogen gas inhalation treatment in acute cerebral infarction: A randomized controlled clinical study on safety and neuroprotection. Journal of Stroke and Cerebrovascular Diseases. 2017;**26**(11):2587-2594

[40] Li TT et al. Molecular hydrogen alleviates lung injury after traumatic brain injury: Pyroptosis and apoptosis. European Journal of Pharmacology. 2022;**914**:174664

[41] Yang WC et al. Molecular hydrogen mediates neurorestorative effects after stroke in diabetic rats: The TLR4/NF-κB inflammatory pathway. Journal of Neuroimmune Pharmacology. 2023;**18**(1-2):90-99

[42] Li TT et al. Effects of a high concentration of hydrogen on neurological function after traumatic brain injury in diabetic rats. Brain Research. 2020;**1730**:146651

[43] Zhou H et al. Hydrogen inhalation decreases lung graft injury in brain-dead donor rats. The Journal of Heart and Lung Transplantation. 2013;**32**(2):251-258

[44] Voet S, Prinz M, van Loo G. Microglia in central nervous system inflammation and multiple sclerosis pathology. Trends in Molecular Medicine. 2019;**25**(2):112-123

[45] Imai K et al. Neuroprotective potential of molecular hydrogen against perinatal brain injury via suppression of activated microglia. Free Radical Biology & Medicine. 2016;**91**:154-163

[46] Chu X et al. Hydrogen-rich saline promotes microglia M2 polarization and complement-mediated synapse loss to restore behavioral deficits following hypoxia-ischemic in neonatal mice via AMPK activation. Journal of Neuroinflammation. 2019;**16**(1):104

[47] Zhuang X et al. Molecular hydrogen attenuates sepsis-induced neuroinflammation through regulation of microglia polarization through an mTOR-autophagy-dependent pathway. International Immunopharmacology. 2020;**81**:106287

[48] Chen H et al. Hydrogen alleviates neuronal injury and neuroinflammation induced by microglial activation via the nuclear factor erythroid 2-related factor 2 pathway in sepsis-associated encephalopathy. Neuroscience. 2021;**466**:87-100

[49] Herzig S, Shaw RJ. AMPK: Guardian of metabolism and mitochondrial homeostasis. Nature Reviews Molecular Cell Biology. 2018;**19**(2):121-135

[50] Jie F et al. Stigmasterol attenuates inflammatory response of microglia via NF-κB and NLRP3 signaling by AMPK activation. Biomedicine & Pharmacotherapy. 2022;**153**:113317

[51] Jiang Y et al. AMP-activated protein kinase links acetyl-CoA homeostasis to BRD4 recruitment in acute myeloid leukemia. Blood. 2019;**134**(24):2183-2194

[52] Fang W et al. Metformin ameliorates stress-induced depression-like behaviors via enhancing the expression of BDNF by activating AMPK/CREB-mediated histone acetylation. Journal of Affective Disorders. 2020;**260**:302-313

[53] Salminen A, Kauppinen A, Kaarniranta K. AMPK/Snf1 signaling regulates histone acetylation: Impact on gene expression and epigenetic functions. Cellular Signalling. 2016;**28**(8):887-895

[54] Wang G et al. HDAC inhibition prevents white matter injury by modulating microglia/macrophage polarization through the GSK3β/PTEN/Akt axis. Proceedings of the National Academy of Sciences of the United States of America. 2015;**112**(9):2853-2858

Section 3

Legal and Emotional Impacts of TBI

Chapter 8

Exploring the Physical and Emotional Damage Legal Proceedings Cause Traumatic Brain Injury Patients

Leighton J. Reynolds

Abstract

This article challenges the current structure regarding legal proceedings with traumatic brain injury cases. Although the legal system most often considers a brain injury to be a single isolated event, that will heal fairly quickly with rest, a traumatic brain injury is more accurately understood as the beginning of a neurodegenerative disease process. The article establishes the neurological and psychological links between stress, brain injuries, and long-term disease. Explores the specific stressors inherent in legal proceedings. And points to the fact that these legal proceedings, which are inherently stressful to begin with, only add further damage to the already fragile health of brain injured persons. The article concludes with strong suggestions regarding how these types of legal cases can be settled more sanely, in a timely manner, and a win-win for everyone. Finally, the author shares his 4 Architecture Model for understanding the neurodegenerative course of a traumatic brain injury with references for further consideration of this model. And how using the "4 Baskets of Symptoms" can help with the diagnosis and treatment of brain injured patients.

Keywords: traumatic brain injuries, concussions, neurodegenerative disease processes, litigation/brain injuries, stress

1. Introduction

Having been involved in legal cases (Workman's Compensation and Personal Injury) over the past 8 years, I have observed the damage that legal proceedings inflict on traumatic brain injury patients. I am writing in the interest of recognizing and changing this fact! The medical and legal perspective I find most often in these cases suggests that concussions involve a single event that will heal, given a few weeks of rest. As Dr. Brent E Masel points out in a ground-breaking article regarding the "standard view" of concussions: "TBI is seen by the insurance industry and many health care providers as an event. For them, once treated and provided with a brief period of rehabilitation, the perception exists that patients with a TBI require little further treatment and face no lasting effects on the CNS or any other organ system in the body." In his view: "TBI increases long-term mortality and reduces life expectancy. TBI are "associated with increased incidences of seizures, sleep disorders, neurodegenerative disorders, neuroendocrine dysregulation and psychiatric diseases, as well as non-neurological disorders such as sexual dysfunction, bladder and bowel incontinence, and systemic metabolic dysregulation that may arise and/or persist for months to years' post-injury" [1].

My experiences with traumatic brain injuries concur with his view. I have observed repeatedly that trauma to the head (at all levels) can be the beginning of a neurodegenerative disease process in the brain over time. In fact, I have never observed an exception to this neurodegenerative disease process following a blow to the head. Sadly, this is too often the beginning of a process that impacts multiple systems in the body and is disease causative and accelerative. Exactly what Dr. Masel was bringing to our attention. In my recently published book, "The Complex Architecture and Healing of Traumatic Brain Injuries: Listening to the Brain" [2]. I present a model of how this deterioration proceeds in the brain/mind, through four interlocking architectures the brain develops in response to being traumatized. These four interlocking architectures are:

Architecture one: shock trauma/traumatic shock.
Architecture two: electrical and chemical disruptions in the brain.
Architecture three: homeostatic breakdown in the mind/brain/body.
Architecture four: the perfect storm in the brain.

(For a detailed description of the four architectures see: "The Complex Architecture and Healing of Traumatic Brain Injuries: Listening to the brain" [2]).

I note further this statement by one of the leading researchers in the world regarding CTE, Dr. Ann C. McKee, that: "All grades of TBI can be associated with long-term physical, emotional, behavioral, and cognitive consequences that permanently affect an individual's ability to perform routine activities and return to work" [3]. Based on my experiences over the past 7 years, I agree with these authors that traumatic brain injuries have long term consequences that need to be addressed. And I would add that brain injuries are not easy to work with because the brain/mind is very complicated, and always involves the person (their developmental history, personality, values, and character) who has the injury. These two issues, the brain injury and the personality who sustained the injury, interact in any treatment situation presenting many complex issues to be dealt with.

Over the past 8 years that I have been working with traumatic brain injury patients I have encountered a lot of resistance to what I am attempting to point out. My credibility has been attacked, I have been accused of creating the patient's illness, and doctors working for the defense have concluded that the plaintiff's current difficulties have nothing to with the concussion or concussions they have suffered. I am challenging current legal proceedings here, because it is my clear and consistent experience that dragging out a legal case is harmful to anyone's health. But it is especially harmful for TBI patients whose health is already very fragile. And my reply is always the same: there is plenty of proof through clinical assessments and brain imaging (Spect scans and fMRIs) that these individuals are struggling with serious disruptions to their normal brain/mind functioning. For a detailed look at these cases see the clinical cases presented in my recent book entitled "The Complex Architecture and Healing of Traumatic Brain Injuries: Listening to The Brain," [2].

Here is what I understand regarding my patients: from healthy, high functioning adult, most working full-time, they now spend much of their time managing deteriorating health, going to a continuous series of doctor's appointments for yet another useless evaluation, while the legal process drags on and on and on. I am very clear that with brain injured patients, demands on the brain, of any kind, take away from the healing process in the brain, and result in even further deterioration of brain functioning. As I point out in my Architecture Model, over time this deteriorating process goes from disruptions in brain/mind functioning to a breakdown of brain/mind functioning. As one of my patients described this deteriorating process: "My brain injury is retarding all my normal responses to life, and this keeps getting worse." This is a serious situation for TBI patients too often unrecognized and hence untreated.

2. Stress and the complex course of a brain injury

Regarding the role stress plays in the lives of victims/patients/clients during their legal proceedings. In my experience the health of the group with the longest exposure to legal proceedings has the most deteriorated medical condition [4]. I also note that the sudden, drastic, and unexpected changes brought about by a brain injury exacerbate the symptoms of stress and mediate poor daily functioning and impaired recovery from the injury. The normal response to stress is worsened after a brain injury as noted below:

In general, TBI patients suffer from a much lower stress tolerance.

They suffer with serious impairments in their ability to evaluate the stressors in their lives.

There is poor initiation and cessation of neuroendocrine stress responses, specifically the role of HPA axis (Hypothalamus-Pituitary-Adrenal).

TBI patients are disproportionately vulnerable to:

- Disease states
- PTSD substance abuse Increased anxiety and depression
- Cardiovascular disease
- Stroke and hemorrhage
- Chronic fatigue and pain
- Cognitive decline
- Sleep disturbances
- Vision and hearing problems
- Serious dissociation (see the neurobiological links between stress, brain injury, and disease [5]).

In addition to the above, the chronic stress of struggling with a traumatic brain injury can alter and damage the Central Nervous System leading to a cascading series of negative outcomes:

Over activation of the neuro-endocrine stress response (HPA axis).
Rising extra-cellular excitatory amino acids (EAA concentrations).
Downstream changes in neuronal structure and function.
Over time then, chronic stress results in permanent alternations in neuroendocrine functioning (HPA axis), the physical structure of the brain, and the individual's behavior.

In summary, I believe medicine, law, and psychology need to understand a TBI as a physical and emotional stressor that produces many parallel physiological and psychological responses: over activation of the HPA stress response axis, inflammatory signals in the body, metabolic dysfunction, excess EAA release, and increases in anxiety, depression, and episodes of dissociation. All of this is directly damaging to the neural structures in the body that mediate the appraisal of physical and psychological threats, and the regulation of neuroendocrine functioning. See The Neurological Effects of Stress on The Brain" [6]: "Left unchecked, there are negative neurological effects of stress on the brain including mental illness, and neurodegenerative diseases like dementia" [7].

The specific stressors TBI patients encounter from our legal system following their injury include:

- Prolonged medical intervention.
- Adapting to a possible prolonged hospitalization.
- Absence from work and when to return.
- Chronic pain.
- Chronic fatigue.
- Disruptions in relationships and family.
- Accumulating new disabilities.
- Disruptions in normal sleep patterns.
- An increase in anxiety and depression.

All the while, the above is superimposed on a nervous system that is impaired in its ability to respond optimally to physical and psychological stressors. TBI patients do not need more stress in their lives such as that which comes along with the legal process.

3. Litigation

Given the above, that a traumatic brain injury is disabling to a person on a wide range of physical and psychological issues, why is the litigation process adding even more stress to an already overtaxed system with all these patients? Look at the list of the increased stressors a TBI person undergoes as a result of the litigation process:

- Finding appropriate medical care.
- Returning to work or not and filling out endless forms.
- Dealing with insurance companies that do not want to pay.
- If a car accident is involved, damage to the vehicle.
- Added burdens to relationships and family.
- The court process itself adding endless (and useless) evaluations, depositions and delays.

All of which can best be understood as Critogenic (law caused) Harm, that is unfortunately intrinsic to the legal process causing inescapable damage to the client/patient both physically and psychologically. This problem is also understood as the "litigation response syndrome." Here complaints arise from the client/patient due solely to the experience of being involved in a lawsuit as opposed to the events that precipitated the injury and the litigation.

In my experience the legal process causes increased stress, anxiety, and depression as the client/patient goes through endless medical evaluations and depositions, repeating and reliving injury details. Sadly, all of this severely impacts the individual's mental, emotional, and physical life. And causes a negative impact on relationships, family and friends. All just when support is most needed as the person struggles with their injury and the legal process.

4. Example

Several years ago, I was involved with a high profile TBI case concerning a NHL player (National Hockey League). Sadly, the medical reports detailing his stressed induced epilepsy were covered up, only coming to light years after his initial concussion and the incident of a Grand Mal Seizure. During the litigation proceedings which dragged on for 7 years, I wrote in my medical reports that further depositions would be detrimental to his health, quite possibly causing him to have another Grand Mal Seizure. Low and behold this is exactly what happened. This incident occurred in November and his case was finally settled the following August.

For me, there are larger issues here such as why it appears that law trumps medicine. I have no doubt that the health of the patient/client should be number one, but in my experience, it is, sadly, not number one by far.

5. Discussion

In doing the research for this chapter, I did come across statements from persons and legal firms that recognized the following: That a traumatic brain injury can significantly impact an individual's competency by affecting cognitive functioning, memory, focus and attention span, judgment, decision making, problem solving (executive functioning), and increase problems with major depression, anxiety and panic attacks, mood swings, behavioral changes and sleep disturbances. These abilities are crucial for understanding and proceeding within the legal system. And it is noted in these articles that proper consideration needs to be given to the unique challenges of TBI patients and the appropriate accommodations they need [8].

There are other articles in the literature that address traumatic brain injuries and the legal process. See:

"Lawsuits and Traumatic Brain Injuries: The Relationship Between Long-Lasting Sequelae and Financial Compensation in Litigants," Results from the Paris-TBI-Study, in Frontiers in Neurology 2019; 10:330 by Eleonore Bayen et al.

"Neuropsychological Aspects of Brain Injury Litigation: A Medicolegal Handbook for Lawyers and Clinicians, Review by Simon F. Crowe in Psychiatry, Psychology and Law 2022; 29 (6): 976-979.

"Understanding Traumatic Brain Injury and It's Legal Implications," by James Schwartz of Schwartz and Schwartz Attorneys at Law, 4/26/2023.

All the above articles address the need for special consideration with traumatic brain injury patients when they are involved in legal proceedings. However, in the 8 years that I have been involved with traumatic brain injuries and I have never seen the court process address what happens in the traumatized brain during the original traumatic event, and what are the consequences of this for brain injured persons. Nor is there any consideration for the individuals who are literally held hostage by the trigger cues that occur long afterward their initial brain injury and are triggered by legal proceedings.

Lastly, I note the following article in Neuro Ethics, "TBI, Neuroscience and The Legal System," [9]. This article explores the role of neuroscience data in the courtroom and suggests addressing the fundamental tension between how the legal system views the causes of behavior and medicine, and how neuroscience and psychology do. Sadly, I have never seen such a discussion in any of the legal cases I have been involved in.

To reiterate, I believe the legal system makes a grave error by not understanding that traumatic brain injuries are always neurodegenerative in nature (different than all other kinds of injuries to the body) and that this is a cascading process in the brain/mind (see the Complex Architecture Model above) that quickly leads to disruptions in brain functioning. If this cascading process in the brain/mind is not treated and healed, then the brain/mind continues its downward course leading to a breaking down in brain/mind functioning and eventually to serious disease processes and illnesses (including Alzheimer's Disease, Parkinson's Disease, Multiple Sclerosis, ALS, CTE, seizures, strokes, and infections). And once again, the stressful processing of legal settlements, by increasing demands on an alright injured brain, push these disease processes forward rather than work to halt them.

6. Conclusion

I do have a suggestion about how these cases can be settled more sanely, in a timely fashion, and a win-win for everyone.

To begin with, I believe all serious blows to the head should be treated in the following manner. An MRI is done immediately to determine if there is any bleeding in the brain, or skull fractures. This should be followed up in the next 2–3 weeks with an fMRI, a functional MRI that looks at the brain in motion, as it is functioning. This is where I see the most damage has occurred. The individual's intelligence will remain intact, and consciousness will remain intact, but it is the execution of intelligence that is so affected. And this situation will deteriorate over time, especially if there is no intervention. Then several months later another fMRI and in 6 months another fMRI to track the neurodegenerative disease process cascading. In my experience, this disease process is always present in one form or another. And this neuro-degenerative process can begin almost immediately following trauma to the brain [10].

As an assessment tool I use the *4 Baskets of Symptoms* which I review with my patients every week:

Physical symptoms (chronic fatigue, chronic pain, difficulty breathing, frequent headaches, frequent migraines, blurred vision, double-vision, tinnitus, frequent urination).

Cognitive decline (brain fog, frequent confusion, declining memory, inability to focus, attend or concentrate, difficulties with judgement and decision making).

Social and emotional Issues (increases in anxiety, depression, dissociation, depersonalization, derealization, and social withdrawal).

Sleep disturbances (loss of normal sleep patterns, insomnia, and the loss of normal, restorative sleep).

Finally, I have found "listening to the brain" (see "The Complex Architecture and Healing of a Traumatic Brain Injury: Listening to the Brain,") [2], and paying close attention to the 4 Baskets of Symptoms (see above), more helpful in the long run than the brain imaging, because it identifies the impairments the patient is struggling with rather than looking only at the diagnosis (which is important in its own way but not sufficient). Working with traumatic brain injuries is difficult, complex, and requires a lot of doctor-patient cooperation. Nonetheless, following the above two guidelines, I have found that traumatic brain injuries can be healed, and patients can return to a normal life.

It is my hope that the above perspective will help to change how TBI cases are processed within the legal system in ways that benefit all.

Author details

Leighton J. Reynolds
Treatment and Tools for Trauma, Los Angeles, CA, United States

*Address all correspondence to: leightonj@sbcglobal.net

References

[1] Masel BE, DeWitt DS. Traumatic brain injury: A disease process, not an event. Neurotrauma. 2010;**27**(8):1529-1540

[2] Reynolds LJ. The Complex Architecture and Healing of Traumatic Brain Injuries. UK: Cambridge Scholars Publishing; 2023

[3] McKee AC, Daneshvar DH. The neuropathology of traumatic brain injury. The Handbook of Clinical Neurology. 2015;**127**:45-66

[4] Clemente M, Padilla-Racero D. The effect of the justice system on mental health. Psychiatry, Psychology, and Law. 2020;**27**(5):856-879

[5] Guo H et al. Neurobiological links between stress, brain injury and disease. Oxidative Medicine and Cellular Longevity. 25 May 2022:8111022

[6] Bouyon P. The Neurological Effects of Stress on the Brain. 2023. Available from: www.inlebrainfitinstitute.com/blog/the-neurological-effects-of-stress-on-the-brain

[7] McEven BS. Neurobiological and Systemic Effects of Chronic Stress. Thousand Oaks: National Library of Congress; Jan-Dec 2017;**1**:2470547017692328

[8] Navigating Traumatic Brain Injury: A Neuropsychological Perspective for the Legal Profession. Available from: www.reflectneuroscience.com

[9] Hardcastle et al. Traumatic brain injury, neuroscience, and the legal system. Neuro Ethics. 2015;**8**:55-64

[10] Reynolds LJ. Listening to the brain/recovering the brain: A case study. SOJ Medical and Clinical Reports. 2023;**3**(2):1-6

Further reading

[11] Saef Izzy MD, Chen PM, Tahir Z, et al. Association of traumatic brain injury with the risk of developing chronic cardiovascular, endocrine, neurological, and psychiatric disorders. JAMA Network Open. 2022;**5**(4):e229478. (Original Investigation Neurology)

[12] Zafonte R. Traumatic brain injury linked to striking 'risk' for CVD, diabetes, and brain disorders. JAMA Network Open. Published online. 2023

[13] Elser H, Gottsman RF, Walton AE. Head injury and long-term mortality risk in community dwelling adults. JAMA Neurology. 2023. Available from: https://pubmed.ncbi.nlm.gov/36689218

Section 4

Rehabilitation and Management of Neurological Conditions

Chapter 9

Management of the Neurogenic Lower Urinary Tract

Thomas Milton, Madeleine Bain and Ashani Couchman

Abstract

Spinal cord injuries commonly impact the complex neurological control of micturition leading to lower urinary tract dysfunction. It can present with lower urinary tract symptoms impacting quality of life, or sequele of incomplete emptying including renal impairment, stones or recurrent infections. It can be classified by location of the injury, however the pattern of symptoms and urodynamics findings may not always directly correlate. Assessment involves a thorough history, examination and investigations, including blood tests, upper tract imaging, bladder diary and urodynamics. Management and ongoing surveillance are tailored to the patient, taking in to account their injury, functional status and trajectory, symptoms and any coexisting bowel or sexual dysfunction. Intermittent catheterisation is the preferred bladder management strategy for incomplete emptying in suitable patients. Anticholinergics and Beta 3 agonists are used for symptoms of overactivity, or alternatively intravesical botulinum toxin injection has been used with high success rates. In select patients, sacral neuromodulation or more complex reconstructions including augmentation or diversion may be required. The overarching goals of treatment are to improve quality of life, maintain social continence, protect the upper tracts and reduce the frequency and severity of infections. This requires a multidisciplinary team to tailor an individualised approach for each patient.

Keywords: spinal cord, neurogenic, dysfunction, urinary tract, management

1. Introduction

The development of neurogenic lower urinary tract dysfunction (NLUTD) following a spinal cord injury (SCI) can have a significant impact on a patients' quality of life, as well as potentially leading to life-threatening complications. 80–90% of patients with SCI will develop some degree of NLUTD [1]. This chapter provides a comprehensive review of the pathophysiology, clinical evaluation and management.

2. Physiology of micturition

Before understanding the pathophysiology of NLUTD in SCI patients, we must first have an understanding of the normal micturition cycle. The micturition cycle is a complex interplay of several structures that are under dynamic neuronal control.

The primary role of the bladder is to store urine until a socially appropriate time to void. The two phases of bladder function, the storage phase and the voiding phase, are dichotomous. The bladder spends 99% of its time in the storage phase and just 1% in the voiding phase [2]. This is just a brief overview of the physiology and for a better understanding, we recommend the use of a dedicated physiology textbook.

2.1 Storage and voiding phase

2.1.1 Storage phase

The bladder is primarily in the storage phase. During this phase, the bladder slowly fills with urine made from the kidneys via both the ureters through the ureteric openings. During filling, the bladder maintains a constant pressure despite the increasing volume, which is referred to as its compliance (change in V/change in P). There are several mechanisms that assist in maintaining its low pressure, including the bladder walls' elastic properties, the smooth muscle's intrinsic ability to maintain a constant tension at different volumes and spinal reflexes that control the detrusor muscle during this phase. When these mechanisms are intact, the bladder is able to store urine at a low pressure. When these mechanisms fail, the pressure in the bladder can overcome that in the ureters leading to reflux of urine, or overcome the urethral sphincter mechanism leading to incontinence.

2.1.2 Voiding phase

In the voiding phase, the bladder and sphincteric mechanisms must do the opposite. Voiding should be efficient so that most of the urine is removed from the bladder. Prior to bladder contraction, the sphincters and pelvic floor relax, creating low pressure in the bladder outlet. Following this, there is contraction of the detrusor muscle, which creates a funnel shape of the bladder neck leading to forceful expulsion of urine out of the internal urethral meatus into the urethra. It is important to note here that during contraction of the detrusor muscle, the distal portion of the ureter which has tunnelled obliquely through the detrusor muscle is constricted, preventing retrograde flow of the urine.

2.1.3 Lower urinary tract symptoms as it relates to bladder physiology

Lower urinary tract symptoms (LUTS) are characterised according to the time that they occur in the micturition cycle, hence when describing LUTS, they can be described as storage LUTS, voiding LUTS or mixed LUTS, which encompasses features of both storage and voiding LUTS. Storage LUTS, which includes urgency, urinary frequency, urge incontinence and altered bladder sensation are indicative of an issue with the storage phase of voiding [3]. Voiding LUTS, which includes hesitancy, intermittency, slow stream, straining and terminal dribbling [3] are due to a problem with the voiding phase, which is most commonly due to bladder outlet obstruction causing an increase in ureteric pressure in the voiding phase.

2.2 Neuronal control

The neuronal control of the bladder involves a complex series of pathways in both the central and peripheral nervous system. It provides coordination of the muscles in the bladder and bladder outlet, receptive relaxation of the bladder, maintains continence with increasing volume in the bladder, sensation of bladder fullness and the initiation of voluntary voiding.

It is under both autonomic and somatic control. The involuntary autonomic control is mediated by sympathetic and parasympathetic pathways and voluntary somatic control by the pudendal nerve. Sympathetic innervation comes from the thoracolumbar outflow and parasympathetic and somatic innervation comes from the sacral segments of the spinal cord. The lower urinary tract is either in its storage phase or voiding phase. During the storage phase, the innervation is under sympathetic control and during the voiding phase it is under parasympathetic control.

In the sympathetic pathway, the postganglionic fibres originate in the T11-L2 spinal cord segments to form the inferior mesenteric ganglia and hypogastric nerve to travel to the bladder and urethra [4]. They release noradrenaline which acts on the bladder and the bladder outlet. In the bladder, noradrenaline activates B3 B-adrenergic inhibitory receptors, resulting in relaxation of the detrusor muscle [5]. In the urethra, noradrenaline activates a-adrenergic excitatory receptors causing contraction of the smooth muscle of the sphincteric mechanism and increasing bladder outlet pressure [4].

In the parasympathetic pathway, postganglionic fibres travel from S2-S4 spinal segments through the pelvic nerves to release acetylcholine (ACh), which effectively has the opposite effect of noradrenaline in the bladder [4]. Acetylcholine targets M3 muscarinic receptors causing contraction of the detrusor muscle and elimination of urine. In the urethra, postganglionic cells release nitric oxide that inhibits their contraction, lowering the pressure in the bladder outlet [4].

The external urethral sphincter is striated muscle under somatic control, allowing it to be voluntarily contracted and relaxed. It is supplied by the pudendal nerve, which may get damaged during parturition. It also releases ACh, resulting in activation of nicotinic receptors and contraction of the external sphincter [4]. The motor neurons controlling this arise from S2-S4 motor neurons in an area called Onuf's nucleus. The pelvic floor is also under somatic control, which is supplied by a motor nucleus at the same spinal level medial to Onuf's nucleus [4].

When the bladder is stimulated or filled, afferent sensory fibres are carried to the spinal cord by pelvic and hypogastric nerves. Bladder distention is carried by A∂ fibres, and noxious stimulus including cooling or irritation is carried by unmyelinated C fibres. These signals are conveyed to S2-4 and T11-L2 spinal segments and communicate both with interneurons in the spinal cord to create spinal reflex arcs and also projecting to higher brain centres [4].

These afferent signals from the filled bladder are integrated at the pontine micturition centre (PMC). The PMC also receives input from multiple higher cortical structures including periaqueductal grey matter (PAG), prefrontal cortex and the hypothalamus that determine whether it is an appropriate time to void [4–6]. During the storage phase, the PMC is inhibited by higher centres. When PMC is inhibited, it leads to activation of sympathetic pathways, and inhibition of parasympathetic pathways. Overall, this causes detrusor relaxation and internal urethral sphincter contraction which allows for filling. When the bladder reaches larger volumes, the afferent signals increase. Higher centres will release their inhibition of PMC. This causes a shift in the balance of autonomic outflow to increase parasympathetic action and decrease sympathetic. This allows contraction of detrusor and voluntary somatic relaxation of the external urethral sphincter.

3. Pathophysiology

Knowledge of the location and extent of a spinal cord injury can provide a theoretical explanation of that patient's neurogenic lower urinary tract dysfunction. However, it should be noted that this is only an association and each patient will present with their own clinical manifestations. There are several reasons that SCI patients have their own unique presentation. Firstly, the SCI may be complete or incomplete, for those that have incomplete SCI, there can be partial transmission of the nervous pathways. Secondly, there will be a variable amount of nervous degeneration and reorganisation distal to the SCI. Thirdly, many patients will have complex SCI with variable degrees of injury at different levels of the spinal cord that are unable to be detected clinically. Regardless, with the current level of understanding of the neuronal control of micturition, the pathophysiology can be described to a degree.

The location of the SCI can be described as suprasacral, sacral/infrasacral or mixed. For suprasacral injuries, or upper motor neuron lesions, communication between the PMC and sacral reflex is disrupted. As the sacral reflex remains intact, the detrusor and external sphincter both become hyperreflexic leading to detrusor overactivity (DO) [5]. The normally coordinated detrusor contraction and sphincter relaxation also becomes disconnected. This leads to simultaneous contraction of both muscles called detrusor sphincter dyssynergia [4]. The loss of compliance of the detrusor muscle and uncoordinated contraction will lead to high intravesical pressures risking damage to the upper tracts [5]. This is effectively a dysfunction of the storage phase of micturition.

A sacral/infrasacral lesion, or a lower motor neuron lesion, will disrupt the sacral reflex arc whilst leaving the PMC intact. Both the detrusor muscle and sphincteric mechanism will be flaccid, hence the detrusor muscle will not contract to void [5]. The pressure remains low in the bladder as its compliance is increased, so the upper tracts are less at risk. When the bladder contains very high volumes of urine, the patient will experience overflow incontinence. This is effectively a dysfunction of the voiding phase of micturition.

Some patients will have an injury that affects the suprasacral area as well as the sacral/infrasacral area. This can encompass dysfunction of both the storage phase and voiding phase of the micturition cycle. The patient may have disruption of the communication pathways of the PMC and sacral reflex and dysfunction of the sacral reflex itself. This can lead to detrusor overactivity or areflexia with increased or reduced bladder compliance. Similarly, the sphincteric mechanism may be hyperreflexic or areflexic, hence these patients may also have DSD. The upper tracts may be at risk if there is reduced bladder compliance and incontinence may occur due to detrusor overactivity or overflow.

4. Classification and aetiology of neurogenic lower urinary tract dysfunction

NLUTD constitutes a vast number of diseases that affect the neurological function of micturition. There are classification systems that exist to assist the clinician to understand the potential clinical consequences for the patient depending on the severity and location of the pathology. Whilst the relationship between the location and severity of disease and the clinical manifestations is not always a direct correlation, it still provides some benefit in predicting the potential outcomes for this patient if their disease is not managed appropriately.

One of the simplest ways to categorise the causes of NLUTD is by the location of the pathology. This can be divided into three or four locations in the central and peripheral nervous system that controls micturition. The four locations are supra-pontine, pontine, suprasacral spinal cord and sacral and subsacral [7]. The European Association of Urology (EAU) guidelines divide the causes into three anatomical locations with multiple sclerosis in its own category called disseminated disease [8].

Unsurprisingly, SCI is located in the spinal region, hence these patients may develop both storage and voiding symptoms, have an elevated PVR and on urodynamics have both DO and DSD. The other causes of spinal pathology may be expected to have a similar presentation in terms of their neuro-urological clinical manifestations but can be easily differentiated on history from SCI patients.

Comprehensive detail on all the causes of NLUTD is beyond the scope of the chapter. This is a list of some of the common causes and their locations:

4.1 Suprapontine lesion

- Cerebrovascular accident
- Brain tumour
- Traumatic head injury
- Dementia
- Parkinson's disease
- Cerebral palsy
- Normal pressure hydrocephalus

4.2 Spinal (infrapontine-suprasacral)

- Spinal cord injury
- Multiple sclerosis
- Spina bifida
- Hereditary spastic paraplegia

4.3 Sacral/infrasacral

- Myelomeningocele
- Spina bifida
- Multiple sclerosis
- Diabetes mellitus
- Iatrogenic

- Lumbar spine degenerative disease
- Lumbar spine disc prolapse
- Lumbar canal stenosis

The level of the SCI can provide further clues as to what clinical manifestations the patient may have. The spinal control of micturition is at S2-S4, hence the level of SCI can be categorised into suprasacral, sacral and infrasacral. Suprasacral lesions can be considered as upper motor neuron lesions, resulting in DO and DSD. Sacral lesions and infrasacral lesions can be considered lower motor neuron lesions, causing detrusor hypo/areflexia and an underactive or denervated external sphincter.

These patterns are not universal and each patient will present with their own spectrum of symptoms. As discussed in pathophysiology, multiple factors influence symptoms including completeness of injury, reorganisation of pathways post injury and complex injuries with variable degrees of dysfunction at different levels of the spinal cord that are unable to be detected clinically.

Perhaps the most useful way to classify NLUTD is based on the results of urodynamics, which will determine the pattern of dysfunction regardless of the anatomical location of the SCI. Clinically, this will be the most beneficial when determining an appropriate management plan for the patient.

5. Evaluation of the neurogenic lower urinary tract disease

There are various guidelines available for the evaluation of NLUTD, (EAU, American Urological Association) however these encompass all causes of NLUTD. Although these guidelines are useful for assessment of this cohort of patients, the evaluation of the SCI patient can be more focused. There are three distinct periods in SCI patients that require different types of evaluation and management, these are the first few weeks after injury, the acute rehabilitation period and lifelong management. In the acute period, the patient requires adequate bladder drainage, with a suprapubic or transurethral catheter until they can safely perform IC. After this period, the patient will require a more comprehensive Urological assessment.

5.1 History and examination

A full history and examination is an essential part of the evaluation. Whilst all components of standard history are important, a thorough discussion focused on the biopsychosocial health of the patient is paramount to determining the most appropriate bladder management strategy and how to support your patient best.

The first part of the history is to characterise their injury. Determine the timing, extent and the mechanism of the injury. The ASIA impairment scale (AIS) score should be documented as part of the assessment of injury. This will help stratify the level of "completeness" of the injury [5].

Both urinary symptoms and their potential complications should be reviewed - including their severity, current management strategies and impact to their quality of life. As discussed earlier in pathophysiology, assess storage symptoms including frequency, urgency, nocturia, incontinence and bladder sensation, as well as voiding symptoms including their stream, intermittency, hesitancy, straining, terminal dribbling or retention. Remember that the presenting LUTS do not necessarily correlate well with the type, extent or level of injury. Complications of urinary tract dysfunction including recurrent infections, renal failure, stone formation should be reviewed. The symptoms may be insidious or vague, but red flags including pain, haematuria or fevers require further investigation [8]. Medications and other medical conditions can also contribute to voiding dysfunction, and it is crucial to recognise other causes for LUTS including bladder outlet obstruction, particularly in older males. Baseline pre-morbid LUTS should be considered. Issues with associated systems often coexist, including bowel and sexual function, and should be included in the assessment [8].

Particular attention should be made to a thorough social and functional history, as this is a strong determinant in which bladder management options are most appropriate. Take note of their dominant hand. The level and degree of injury influences hand fine motor function, mobility, transfers and their overall functional outcomes. Consider not only their current functional status, but also the likely trajectory of their functional status which may change over time. Social factors including their support network, home setup and equipment, financial circumstances and impact to employment, cultural or spiritual beliefs and whether they have close and easy access to specialised healthcare also strongly influences what additional supports are required.

The physical assessment should include examination of the abdomen and external genitalia, neurological system and digital rectal exam. Rectal tone, presence of the bulbocavernosus reflex or sphincter contraction should be assessed [5]. Patient quality of life questionnaires can be used to evaluate the effect of treatment and is an essential component to consider in management. Multiple questionnaires exist, but the one chosen should be validated in the neuro-urological population and take into account the patients' literacy and primary language [8].

5.2 Investigations

Unfortunately, the bladder tends to be an unreliable witness due to multiple factors. These include subjective bias from the patient history, the significant overlap of symptoms between different conditions, the existence of multiple conditions that influence LUTS and the poor correlation between the extent/level of the SCI and LUTS.

There are simple, non-invasive tests that the majority of patients will initially have which include bedside assessments, blood tests and imaging. If an answer from these tests is provided, they will not need to progress to more invasive testing, however the vast majority of patients with a SCI will require more invasive investigations. The invasive tests will have to be rationalised based on the injury and impairment level.

Urodynamics is an umbrella term that includes several non-invasive and invasive investigations. It includes: a post-void residual, voiding diary, pad testing, uroflowmetry, pressure/flow studies and video urodynamics. The aim of urodynamic testing is to reproduce the patient's LUTS and provide an objective analysis of this. This will provide a precise diagnosis and dictate further management. It should be noted here that in clinical practice, the term urodynamics is often used to refer to cystometry with or without video urodynamics.

The underlying principles of urodynamic evaluation is to reproduce the patients' abnormalities in the micturition cycle to provide an objective and pathophysiology explanation for their symptoms. The correct study needs to be chosen to reproduce the symptoms to provide an answer. For this reason, urodynamics can only be properly evaluated when there is accompanying clinical information for correlation.

5.3 Blood tests and imaging

Baseline biochemistry and imaging form part of the assessment, especially to screen for any complications that have arisen from incomplete emptying. Blood tests for renal function should be done as a baseline and can be monitored to signal evolving renal impairment [8].

Ultrasound imaging of the renal tract is used to assess the upper tracts for hydroureter, the bladder for post void residual (PVR) as well as assessing for any coexisting urological issues including prostatomegaly [8]. This should be included as part of the initial assessment, and the frequency of ongoing upper tract surveillance is based on the patients risk of developing high bladder pressures, reflux and renal impairment [5].

5.4 Non-invasive urodynamics

5.4.1 Post-void residual

A simple yet extremely useful test. It can be done in any clinical setting in which a bladder scanner or ultrasound is available or an in and out catheter at the end of a spontaneous void. However, this requires voluntary control over voiding, which is likely impaired in the SCI patient.

PVR is variable for each patient and will increase in the elderly. There is a lack of consensus for absolute cut off values, however it is generally accepted that a PVR of less than 50 mL is considered normal [9]. A PVR of >200–300 mL or 30% of the voided volume suggests dysfunction of bladder emptying and may be significant [9, 10]. It is important to note that these numbers can be deceiving. The true assessment of the significance of a PVR requires a voided volume for comparison. An elevated PVR may be due to detrusor underactivity, bladder outlet obstruction or rarely a combination of both. An elevated PVR could indicate acute or chronic urinary retention and is an indication for prostate-reductive surgery in males with bladder outlet obstruction. An elevated PVR is considered a risk factor for recurrent UTIs [9]. It may also be associated with hydronephrosis which may indicate a high pressure system, and this would ideally prompt further evaluation with formal urodynamics or effective bladder emptying either by utilising clean intermittent catheterisation or indwelling catheterisation.

5.4.2 Bladder diary

Another simple and extremely useful test. For the most meaningful results, it requires a motivated patient who is willing to do the bladder diary at home prior to the consultation. It gives objective evidence of the patient's voiding pattern and demonstrates the severity and impact on the patient's life. Over a 3-day period, the patient should record when they go to sleep, when they wake up, fluid intake, time of void, volume of void and include a comments section to mention sensations of urgency or episodes of incontinence [8]. An example of a bladder diary is provided below and patient instructions is provided (**Figure 1**).

In SCI patients, a voiding diary will not always be possible. It is can be useful if the patient is performing IC and redundant if they have an in-dwelling catheter. Regardless, in patients that can do a bladder diary, a pattern of voiding can be determined. For example, in patients who void frequently with low volumes and document a sense of urgency and urge incontinence, this points towards a diagnosis of detrusor overactivity. It may demonstrate the patient has urinary frequency with normal

DOI: http://dx.doi.org/10.5772/intechopen.1006148

a)

Input/Output Day One

Time	Type	In	Out	Wet

b)

This "bladder diary" is used to assess how much fluid you drink, to measure your urine you make, to record how often you pass urine over 24 hours and to show any episodes of urine leak.

You should fill in the chart as accurately as possible over three days.

You will need a measuring jug to measure the urine you pass. You could measure how much your cup holds to make it easier to estimate how much you are drinking.

Every time you have a drink, make a note of how much it is (in mL if possible) and enter this value in the "IN" column and note the time. Try to record every drink, day and night. Record the type of drink (water, squash, coffee, tea, beer etc) in the "TYPE" column because this can help us identify any triggers for your symptoms.

Each time you pass urine, collect it in your measuring jug, measure the amount (in mL, if possible) and record it in the "OUT" column and note the time. If, for any reason, you are not able to measure how much urine you have passed, simply put a tick in the appropriate "OUT" box.

If you have any urine leakage by night or day, mark the box under the column heading "WET" against the appropriate time slot. You can add mild, moderate of severe.

Figure 1.
(a) An example of a bladder diary for patient to complete, and (b) the instructions provided to the patient.

volumes being voided, which may be associated with high fluid intake or diabetes mellitus. It is a crucial tool to diagnose nocturnal polyuria which is the excessive and disproportionate excretion of urine during the patients main sleep period [11]. It is often expressed as a proportion of the 24 hour voided volume, and is said to be present if nocturnal output is >20% of the total in younger patients and > 33% in those >65 years old [11]. If there is incontinence, it can be useful adjunct to assess volume of incontinence and can be further supported by pad weights. And of course, it may show the patient is voiding at a normal frequency with normal volumes.

5.5 Invasive urodynamics

As mentioned above, urodynamics refers to all investigations that objectively demonstrate the function of the lower urinary tract. However, in practice, albeit incorrectly, the term urodynamics is primary used to describe pressure/flow cystometry. The benefit of this study is that it provides simultaneous information on bladder pressures and voiding function so that the precise site of dysfunction can be determined. The most important urodynamic assessment in SCI patients is cystometry, which measures the pressure in the bladder during the micturition cycle. Video urodynamics is the gold standard, but is not always readily available. Some patients will also require a flexible cystoscopy to supplement urodynamic evaluation.

It is important that correct terminology is used when describing urodynamics. As described in the micturition cycle above, the bladder and urethra must be coordinated to have appropriate voiding function and continence. During the storage phase, the bladder should be relaxed and the urethra active. During filling in cystometry, the bladder and urethra should be described as active or underactive. If the bladder pressure is higher than expected during the filling phase, this may be due to detrusor overactivity or if sustained, due to poor compliance of the bladder. If the urethra pressure is low during the storage phase, this represents an incompetent urethral sphincter. Conversely, during the voiding phase, the detrusor should be active and urethra relaxed. If the pressure is lower than expected in the bladder, this represents detrusor underactivity. If the pressure is high in the urethra during contraction of the detrusor, this represents detrusor-sphincter dyssynergia.

Sensation is also recorded for degrees of subjective fullness. It can be normal, oversensitive, reduced or absent, or other abnormal sensations including tingling, non-specific awareness or pain [3].

5.5.1 Common findings in SCI patients

- Detrusor overactivity (thoracic SCI)
- Detrusor-sphincter dyssynergia (thoracic SCI)
- Detrusor underactivity (sacral SCI)
- Sensory deficit

5.6 Common presentations of NLUTD

There are multiple possible ways in which a patient with a spinal cord injury may present with NLUTD. As discussed above, this is influenced by many factors including the level and severity of injury, any coexisting pathology and whether complications have developed. Some of the common presentations are spinal shock, urinary retention, urinary incontinence, recurrent UTIs and deteriorating renal function.

Injuries at a suprasacral level will typically have storage dysfunction due to detrusor overactivity and DSD as they lose the higher control from PMC and rely on spinal reflexes. Patients may present with bothersome incontinence, frequency and urgency. If Detrusor sphincter dyssynergia (DSD) is significant they may also have hesitancy, an interrupted stream and need for double voiding or the inability to generate a void. The urodynamic findings which support this are an increase in detrusor pressure, the filling of the proximal urethra and closure of the sphincter complex. Fluoroscopic views demonstrate the classic finding of a "goblet" shape with attenuation of the column of contrast at the sphincter with minimal onward passage. Bladder pressures during urodynamics are crucial to stratify risk of upper tract in this patient group.

These patients are more likely to develop upper tract complications as a result of higher pressures, which is defined as bladder pressures in excess of 40cmH2O (DLPP >40cmH2)) with a subsequent impairment of upper tract anatomy (hydronephrosis and attenuation of renal parenchyma) and renal function.

The aetiology of voiding dysfunction in sacral/infra sacral injuries is considered to be the impairment of the spinal voiding reflexes. This produces decreased detrusor contraction and may have impaired sphincter contraction leading to a large, poorly contractile bladder [3]. They can present with incontinence, which is typically as a result of overflow. Post void residuals are elevated and urodynamics features include poor detrusor contraction on voiding with a large compliant/"hypercompliant" bladder. The urethral sphincter can be normoactive or under active. As these patients maintain lower bladder pressures due to increased compliance, they tend to have a lower risk of upper tract complications than those with higher injuries. Mixed upper motor and lower motor neuron lesions can present with any constellation of the above findings.

Patients can also present with the complications of their voiding dysfunction. Urinary tract infections are common complications in spinal cord injury patients irrespective of what bladder management strategy they choose. They can present with multiple possible local symptoms including pyuria, new incontinence, pain or pressure, or systemic symptoms including fevers, malaise, anorexia, spasms or autonomic dysreflexia. Recurrent or relapsing infections can signal incomplete bladder emptying or a structural abnormality as a contributing cause. Foreign bodies, bladder stones or tumours can become a nidus for infection and should be excluded [2]. Technique and hygiene should also be assessed as a potential modifiable factor. Deteriorating renal function can have a myriad of causes. In the spinal cord injury patient, a full assessment including PVR and urodynamics can assess whether there is a post renal cause due to high intravesical pressures or incomplete emptying.

6. Management of neurogenic lower urinary tract dysfunction

The management of these patients requires a personalised approach. The key treatment goals are to attain social continence, protect upper tracts, maintain the renal function and reduce the frequency and severity of UTIs [8]. However, each patient may have their own personal treatment goals and the care provided should be individualised. A conservative management approach is the preferred option, as it gives the patient the best opportunity to continue their life with a degree of normalcy. A conservative approach includes regular counselling, lifestyle/behavioural changes, adequate bladder emptying, pharmacological management and annual surveillance. As the patient ages, their pathology progresses or they develop other conditions contributing to LUTS, their targeted management plan should be adapted to meet their requirements. If there are signs that a conservative approach is not sufficient, such as incontinence, recurrent UTIs or deteriorating renal function, the patient may require more invasive management options. A flow diagram of the management is shown below. This section will discuss the conservative management approach, operative options and management of UTIs (**Figure 2**).

6.1 Conservative management

Whenever possible, conservative management is the best option to start the treatment journey. In the acute phase of recovery following a traumatic spinal cord

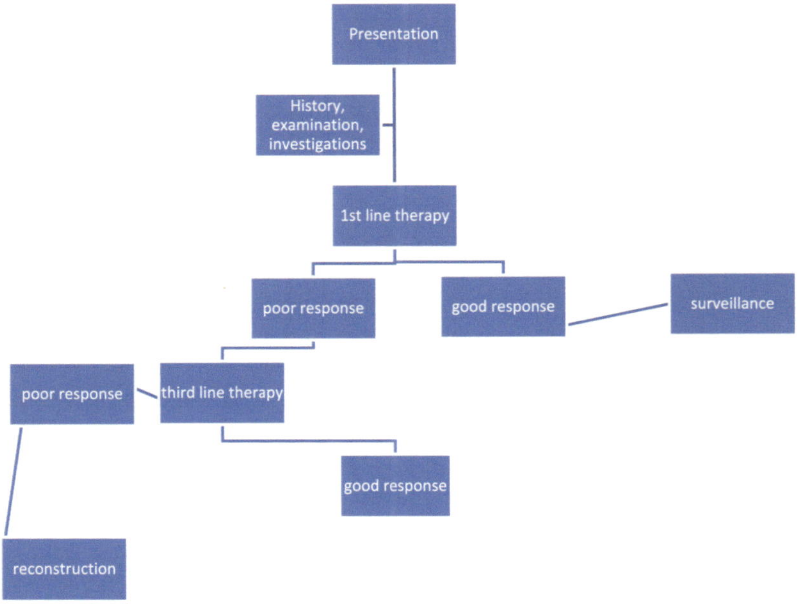

Figure 2.
Treatment algorithm.

injury in patients who are unable to void, a permanent catheter should be placed for adequate bladder emptying. Certain centres advocate the early utilisation of intermittent catheterisation often by a third party. This approach will depend on the skill, resources and equipment available to the unit. The patient should be given the opportunity to spontaneously void after they have recovered from the acute phase. Further investigation should be delayed until after the acute phase, so that their neurological deficits can be assessed to guide long-term management.

When commencing management, the first component is to determine some key aspects about the patient that will impact whether or not they are suitable for conservative measures. Take note of the patient's level and extent of SCI and make an assessment of their underlying neurological function. The patients' age, cognitive status, hand dexterity, hand dominance and mobility will impact their ability to empty their bladder safely. It should also be considered if the patient has any other medical conditions that may impact their bladder emptying, such as bladder outlet obstruction, cardiac failure and subsequent diuretic use, diabetes mellitus and metabolic syndrome.

An important aspect of this patient cohort to consider is the impact on the patients sexual function and fertility. Patients require appropriate counselling on this as it can significantly impact their quality of life. Male patients can have altered ejaculation and erectile function, which may affect fertility. For erections, medications such as phosphodiesterase5-inhibitors, which can be given orally or as an intracavernosal injection. If there is not success with medications, external pumps or a penile prosthesis can be used. Female patients may also experience an altered orgasm as well.

Bladder emptying is an important element of the management of these patients. For patients unable to spontaneously void safely, their options for bladder emptying are intermittent catheterisation (IC), indwelling urethral catheter (IDC) or suprapubic catheter (SPC). The preferred option is IC, as not only does this reduce the risk of UTIs, it also allows patients to be more comfortable in social settings [8]. Unfortunately, not all patients will be appropriate for IC, such as patients with cognitive deficits without bladder sensation who may not remember to perform IC, severe neurological deficits or arthritis affecting their dexterity, disorders of vision, anatomical issues such as obesity or a buried penis and finally patient preference. If unable to perform IC, an IDC or SPC must be placed. These both carry similar risks of UTI. The preference is for an SPC when possible, to allow for easier catheter changes, prevent urethral erosion or bladder neck dilation from a urethral catheter. An SPC may not be possible for all patients, such as patients who have had extensive previous abdominal surgery, bladder cancer or obesity. For selected patients with urinary incontinence, a urodome may be an option if it can be applied anatomically.

Bladder storage impairment should concomitantly managed. In detrusor overactivity, the recommendations must include modification of fluid intake if appropriate, reducing caffeine and carbonated drinks. The use of pelvic floor exercises and bladder retraining can be helpful, as well as vaginal oestrogen cream or pessary. A bowel management program should be in place to assist in overall management.

Pharmacological therapies can then be introduced as second-line treatment. Medications for storage LUTS include anticholinergics and beta-3 agonists. The medication chosen should be a shared decision between the clinician and the patient. Local pharmaceutical benefit schemes should be reviewed for the cost of each medication, as this may influence which option is feasible for the patient. If there is no improvement with one medication, another within the same class should be considered as an alternative. The patient should be counselled on possible adverse effects, such as dry mouth, constipation, retention and cognitive decline in the case of antimuscarinic therapy. The mechanism of an anticholinergic is to competitively inhibit the muscarinic receptors that acetylcholine targets, leading to relaxation of the detrusor muscle. If there is no improvement on an anticholinergic, a beta-3 agonist, such as mirabegron, can be either used with or instead of an anticholinergic. Mirabegron targets beta receptors in the bladder leading to detrusor relaxation. The most important adverse effect is hypertension, and the patient should have their blood pressure monitored, with cessation of mirabegron if they become hypertensive.

6.2 Operative management

Third-line options consist of surgical management of varying degrees of invasiveness. These options include Botox administration, sacral neuromodulation, percutaneous tibial nerve stimulation, mid-urethral slings, artificial urinary sphincters and urethral bulking agents [2, 5, 8].

Neurogenic detrusor overactivity dry/wet can be managed well with intravesical botulinum toxin administered under local anaesthetic or under sedation. Success rates are quoted as >90% in this cohort and is a robust and safe option in the long term [12]. Botulinum toxin is a toxin extracted from the bacteria Clostridium Botulinum. The toxin works by decreasing the release of acetylcholine at the neuromuscular junction, therefore reducing muscle contraction. This is a reversible process, with the effects being variable for each patient, with an estimated effect of 9 months [5]. The introduction of this therapy has reduced the need for further surgical intervention in the modern management of neurogenic detrusor overactivity. Systematic instillation of Botox into the bladder is administered in several injections to the base of the bladder carefully avoiding administration into the trigone or near the ureteric openings. However, there is heterogeneity of botulinum toxin delivery with no clear template demonstrably better than another. Patients will have a variable response to the dose as well and will require titration with each injection. For patients who do not have a permanent catheter, they are at an increased risk of urinary retention in the post-operative period and must be educated on performing IC prior to being given Botox [13]. This procedure may also cause autonomic dysreflexia in SCI patients with injuries T8 and above. For these patients, Botox should be administered with anaesthetic support and monitoring, as well as prophylactic antihypertensives for those with a history of autonomic dysreflexia.

Sacral neuromodulation is postulated as a minimally invasive therapy that is increasing in its utilisation. It has the advantage of not impairing voiding function and can be attractive to patients who do not want to be exposed to the risk of detrusor failure that Botulinum toxin can afford. The postulated mechanisms include activation of C fibre pathways, activation of sacral voiding reflexes or dampening guarding reflexes. With the advent of MRI compatible leads with the associated benefit of improved bowel function, there is an increase in the utilisation of this therapy particularly in the MS population of ambulant patients. A pulse generator is inserted in the upper outer quadrant on the same side as the patients' dominant hand. A test stimulator is used prior to surgery to determine if the patient has any response to neuromodulation. The disadvantage of SNM, is that the patient must have reasonable hand function, cognition and mobility to be able to operate the device. The battery life varies depending on the manufacturer from 10 to 15 years, hence will require to be changed periodically.

Percutaneous tibial nerve stimulation can be helpful in this presentation, but success rates are variable and less effective than botulinum toxin or sacral neuromodulation. Emerging therapies including intracranial stimulation have been described but are not in use outside research settings.

In cases of concomitant stress incontinence, the volume of incontinence will dictate the therapy. Pelvic floor exercises are difficult with poor recruitment of muscles, poor sensation and in the case of some patients, previous pelvic trauma scarring the pelvic floor and impairment of pelvic nerve function. Biofeedback can be a useful adjunct in this setting, usually undertaken by skilled physiotherapists. To supplement this in low volume stress incontinence, urethral bulking can be a robust and repeatable, low impact procedure. With the advent of hyaluronic acid derivatives, the risk of erosion and migration is mitigated to a degree, and is well tolerated in patients injected by an experienced surgeon. In moderate incontinence, a number of adjunctive devices/artificial slings can be considered. However, in this population with an increased risk of erosion and high likelihood of concomitant IC, it would be prudent to be thoughtful in considering insertion. Artificial urinary sphincters placed either at the bulbar urethra, transcorporal or around the bladder neck can be an excellent option for high volume incontinence. The well placed fascial sling in either gender can be a well tolerated safe procedure to increase outlet resistance. The final option of bladder neck closure should not be considered unless all other options have been exhausted as this can impair emergency access to the bladder increasing the risk to the patient.

In the motivated patient, alternative reconstructive options remain available. Mitrofanoff formation, augmentation cystoplasty or ileal conduit diversion remain options to support continence and self-management of the urinary tract while reducing the risk of upper tract compromise. These procedures must be part of the armamentarium of the Neuro-Urologist to ensure that a complete management plan can be delivered through the lifetime of bladder evolution in this patient population.

6.3 UTI management

The management of UTIs in SCI patients poses many challenges as they are common, initially subtle or atypical in presentation and can rapidly deteriorate. It is a crucial part of their management as this group is at a higher risk of complications, such as pyelonephritis, renal damage, urosepsis and death, as well as the risk of autonomic dysreflexia in patients with a SCI above T6. There are several factors that increase the complexity of their management, including the use of catheters, incomplete emptying of their bladders, overtreatment of asymptomatic bacteriuria and subsequent multidrug resistant organisms. When SCI patients present unwell, there should be a high index of suspicion that it may be due to a UTI, as they can present with atypical or vague symptoms.

When managing recurrent UTIs, it is important to use local practices protocols. A urine dipstick is often inaccurate and a urine culture may miss a significant number of infections, and conversely, a positive urine culture is often due to contamination [14]. For some patients, the best tool for diagnosing a UTI is a clinician who is familiar with the patient with a good rapport who can detect the patients' unique symptoms when they have a UTI.

The frequent use of antibiotics when not required can lead to the occurrence of multi-drug resistant organisms, which are more difficult to treat. The guidelines for treatment of UTIs will continue to evolve as new drug-resistant organisms arise and guidelines should be continually updated as new evidence emerges. There is much debate over the use of long-term, low-dose prophylactic antibiotics in these patients, which should follow local guidelines.

Adjunctive therapies such as D-mannose, Hiprex with Vitamin C, UTI vaccines and intravesical antibiotic therapy can be utilised in selected patients with good effect. Good bowel management should be advocated with every patient in the holistic management of recurrent UTI. Supportive allied health professionals are also key in the interdisciplinary care.

6.4 Surveillance

Long term management of SCI patients requires a multidisciplinary care approach. The follow-up of these patients is variable and should follow local practices. For high-risk patients who are stable, annual follow-up is advised with upper tract imaging and renal function evaluation [5, 8]. These follow-ups review the patients LUTS, frequency of UTIs, presence of stones, upper tract dilatation and renal function, which may be a sign the patient requires adjustment to their management plan. The presence of bladder stones may be a sign that the patient is inadequately emptying their bladder.

6.5 Autonomic dysreflexia

Patients with SCIs at T6 and above are at risk of developing autonomic dysreflexia. Autonomic dysreflexia is an exaggerated sympathetic response due to a stimulus below the level of the SCI. Possible stimuli include UTIs, bladder stones, urinary retention and urological procedures such as catheter insertion, cystoscopy and urodynamics. The patient will develop severe hypertension, headaches, sweating and bradycardia. This should be treated as an emergency. The patient will require blood pressure monitoring and treatment such as a GTN patch. The causative stimulus should be removed or treated. Patients who have had autonomic dysreflexia should be counselled on the symptoms so that they can seek medical attention urgently in the future.

7. Conclusion

The urologist is a key member in the multidisciplinary team to provide both acute care and lifelong surveillance in spinal cord injury patients. As circumstances evolve over time, conservative, pharmacological and surgical options should be utilised from the armamentarium of management strategies to create an individualised approach for the patient.

Conflict of interest

The authors declare no conflict of interest.

Author details

Thomas Milton[1*], Madeleine Bain[2] and Ashani Couchman[1]

1 Royal Adelaide Hospital, Adelaide, Australia

2 Redcliffe Hospital, Brisbane, Australia

*Address all correspondence to: thomas.milton@health.sa.gov.au

References

[1] Weld KJ, Dmochowski RR. Association of level of injury and bladder behavior in patients with post-traumatic spinal cord injury. Urology. 2000;**55**(4):490-494

[2] Panicker JN. Neurogenic bladder: Epidemiology, diagnosis, and management. Seminars in Neurology. 2020;**40**(5):569-579

[3] Gajewski JB, Schurch B, Hamid R, Averbeck M, Sakakibara R, Agrò EF, et al. An international continence society (ICS) report on the terminology for adult neurogenic lower urinary tract dysfunction (ANLUTD). Neurourology and Urodynamics. 2018;**37**(3):1152-1161

[4] Fowler CJ, Griffiths D, de Groat WC. The neural control of micturition. Nature Reviews. Neuroscience. 2008;**9**(6):453-466

[5] Perez NE, Godbole NP, Amin K, Syan R, Gater DR. Neurogenic bladder physiology, pathogenesis, and management after spinal cord injury. Journal of Personalized Medicine. 2022;**12**(6)

[6] Gajewski JB, Drake MJ. Neurological lower urinary tract dysfunction essential terminology. Neurourology and Urodynamics. 2018;**37**(S6):S25-S31

[7] Chapple CR, Hillary CJ, Patel A, SA MD. Urodynamics Made Easy. 4th ed. Great Britain: Elsevier; 2018

[8] Neuro-urology [Internet]. EAU Guidelines Office, Arnhem, The Netherlands: EAU Guidelines. 2024. [Updated 2024; cited 2024 Jun 15]. Available from: https://uroweb.org/guidelines

[9] Asimakopoulos AD, De Nunzio C, Kocjancic E, Tubaro A, Rosier PF, Finazzi-Agrò E. Measurement of post-void residual urine. Neurourology and Urodynamics. 2016;**35**(1):55-57

[10] Alagiakrishnan K, Valpreda M. Ultrasound bladder scanner presents falsely elevated postvoid residual volumes. Canadian Family Physician. 2009;**55**(2):163-164

[11] Hashim H, Blanker MH, Drake MJ, Djurhuus JC, Meijlink J, Morris V, et al. International continence society (ICS) report on the terminology for nocturia and nocturnal lower urinary tract function. Neurourology and Urodynamics. 2019;**38**(2):499-508

[12] Kuo H-C. Therapeutic effects of suburothelial injection of botulinum a toxin for neurogenic detrusor overactivity due to chronic cerebrovascular accident and spinal cord lesions. Urology. 2006;**67**(2):232-236

[13] Cruz F, Herschorn S, Aliotta P, Brin M, Thompson C, Lam W, et al. Efficacy and safety of onabotulinumtoxinA in patients with urinary incontinence due to neurogenic detrusor overactivity: A randomised, double-blind, placebo-controlled trial. European Urology. 2011;**60**(4):742-750

[14] Hoffman JM, Wadhwani R, Kelly E, Dixit B, Cardenas DD. Nitrite and leukocyte dipstick testing for urinary tract infection in individuals with spinal cord injury. The Journal of Spinal Cord Medicine. 2004;**27**(2):128-132

Chapter 10

Rehabilitation of Spinal Cord Injury

Zeynep Karakuzu Güngör

Abstract

Spinal cord injury (SCI) involves damage to the spinal cord, extending from the foramen magnum to the cauda equina, resulting from either traumatic or nontraumatic causes. The extent of functional impairment is closely associated with whether the injury is categorized as complete or incomplete, as well as its specific level. SCI exerts a multi-systemic impact on patients, leading to various complications including orthostatic hypotension, autonomic dysreflexia, neurogenic bladder, neurogenic bowel dysfunction, urinary tract infections, pressure ulcers, fractures, deep vein thrombosis, spasticity, heterotopic ossification, contractures, and pulmonary and cardiovascular issues, in addition to depressive disorders. Timely initiation of rehabilitation plays a pivotal role in fostering patient independence and averting potential complications post-SCI. Employing an interdisciplinary approach is imperative in SCI rehabilitation due to its multifaceted nature. The rehabilitation journey following SCI is protracted and arduous, necessitating both the patient's resilience and motivation. Our decision has been made to conduct a comprehensive review encompassing all facets of rehabilitation for SCI patients.

Keywords: spinal cord injury, rehabilitation, physical therapy, neurological rehabilitation, interdisciplinary care

1. Introduction

Spinal cord injury (SCI) represents a sudden and enduring neurological condition associated with substantial morbidity and mortality throughout an individual's lifetime [1]. The etiology of SCI can be categorized into two main groups: traumatic and nontraumatic. Traumatic SCI typically results from significant trauma, such as traffic accidents, falls, or violence, while nontraumatic causes encompass infections, inflammatory myelitis, vascular or noninflammatory myelopathies, various tumors, or congenital anomalies. This manuscript primarily focuses on traumatic SCI due to its prevalence and distinct characteristics [2, 3].

SCI constitutes a formidable medical challenge, marked by a high incidence of disability and mortality [4]. Globally, there are over 27 million individuals living with SCI, with approximately one million new cases emerging annually, with falls and motor vehicle accidents being the primary causes [5]. Notably, there's a rising trend of SCI affecting younger individuals, predominantly under 30 years of age

IntechOpen

[6]. The irreversible motor and sensory deficits ensuing SCI have profound implications for affected individuals, often leading to higher rates of depression or anxiety compared to the general population [7–9]. Moreover, the financial burden per SCI patient is typically substantial [10], encompassing physical, psychological, and financial domains.

Despite advancements, the precise pathological mechanisms underlying spinal cord injury (SCI) remain complex and undefined, necessitating clinical diagnosis primarily through physical examination, imaging techniques, and relevant biochemical markers [11]. SCI is broadly categorized as either complete or incomplete, with complete SCI characterized by the absence of preserved motor or sensory function below the level of injury [12]. Depending on the level of the lesion, SCI can present as paraplegia (impairing only the lower limbs) or tetraplegia/quadriplegia, affecting sensory and motor function in all four limbs. It is crucial to note that management approaches vary according to the completeness and level of the lesion [12]. Systematic reviews suggest no significant disparity in frequency between complete and incomplete SCI or between paraplegia and tetraplegia, although such trends may differ between developed and developing nations [13, 14]. Despite recent progress, individuals with SCI continue to face an elevated risk of mortality, especially during the early stages following trauma [15].

As a result of trauma, important psychological, physiological, and social problems are experienced. In the past, SCI was seen as an incurable disease for many years, but in parallel with the developments in medicine in the twentieth centuries, the survival rates and life spans of patients have gradually increased and approached the values of normal society. The aim of spinal cord injury rehabilitation is to maximize physical independence, improve quality of life and make the patient a productive individual who undertakes age-appropriate social roles. Determining the patient's expectations and achievable goals significantly affects the motivation for follow-up and treatment. With early rehabilitation, acute complications can be prevented and it is easier to achieve functional gains in the chronic period. Rehabilitation is an interdisciplinary teamwork; the leader of the team is the physiatrist. Other members of the team are the patient and his/her family, physiotherapist, occupational therapist, nurse, social worker, orthotist, dietician, specialist physicians from other branches (such as an orthopedist, neurosurgeon, urologist, plastic surgeon, internal medicine specialist, psychiatrist). In addition, respiratory therapists and speech therapists can be added when necessary. Patients treated in special SCI units are reported to have higher survival rates, fewer complications, shorter hospitalization periods and better rehabilitation outcomes [16].

Rehabilitation is expected to be more satisfactory with a team trained and experienced in the care of patients with SCI. Early rehabilitation after injury is very important for the person's adaptation to life and achieving the goals set.

2. Classification

The functional status of individuals with spinal cord injury (SCI) is intricately tied to the type and level of injury sustained. Complete injury results in a complete loss of motor and sensory functions beyond the injury site. In contrast, incomplete injury involves partial preservation of sensory and motor functions below the neurological level, including the lower sacral segments, allowing for the retention of deep anal sensation and/or superficial anal mucocutaneous sense. The determination of lesion status remains uncertain until the conclusion of the spinal shock period, with an increase in reflex activity serving as a positive indicator, despite ongoing debates regarding definitive signs marking the end of this period.

The classification of spinal cord injuries is established by the American Spinal Injury Association (ASIA) based on motor and sensory functions. In the 2011 revision of the ASIA Impairment Scale, the term "deep anal pressure" replaced "deep anal sense". However, in the latest iteration of the International Standards for Neurological Classification of Spinal Cord Injury (ISNCSC), the concept of skeletal level is omitted [17, 18].

The ASIA Impairment Scale categorizes spinal cord injuries as follows:

A. Complete injury, where no motor or sensory function is retained in the sacral segments S4–S5.

B. Incomplete injury, characterized by preserved sensory but not motor function below the neurological level, encompassing the sacral segments S4–S5.

C. Incomplete injury, with preserved motor function below the neurological level, where more than half of key muscles below that level exhibit a muscle grade less than three.

D. Incomplete injury, featuring preserved motor function below the neurological level, with at least half of key muscles below that level demonstrating a muscle grade of three or higher.

E. Normal function.

3. Mechanism of injury

The natural progression of spinal cord injury (SCI) comprises two principal phases: primary injury and secondary injury. Primary injury results from the direct damaging impact of the causative agent on the spinal cord tissue, whereas secondary injury ensues from subsequent events following neural tissue damage and the infiltration of immune-inflammatory cells into the injured area [19]. Primary injury is typically irreversible and occurs abruptly, often with unpredictable outcomes, while secondary injury may exhibit a delayed onset.

Clinically, secondary injury can be delineated into acute (minutes to hours), subacute (hours to 3–4 months), and chronic (months to years) phases. During these phases, SCI patients may experience distinct phenomena such as spinal shock, lasting 8–12 weeks, neurogenic shock, persisting for 3–4 months, and immunoinflammatory shock, spanning 1–4 months [20–22].

4. Rehabilitation

4.1 Acute period

After stabilization of the spine, acute care units/rehabilitation in patients referred to intensive care units the process begins. Neurological examinations of the patients are carried out in detail the presence of early complications or risk is assessed. Secondary rehabilitation in early rehabilitation prevents complications, accelerates neural recovery and injury maximizing functional status after target.

After the examination of the patient, the evaluation is completed with laboratory and imaging methods. These include routine biochemical tests, urine culture, wound or ostomy culture, chest and injury radiographs, and pulmonary function tests in upper-level injuries.

In addition, urodynamics, venous Doppler ultrasonography, tomography, or magnetic resonance imaging is performed when necessary, and may be requested.

After these evaluations are completed, the most appropriate rehabilitation program for the patient is prepared and implemented by the rehabilitation team.

The most important condition in early rehabilitation is positioning. The appropriate position for bed is defined as hip and knees in extension and feet and ankles in 900 dorsiflexion position. To prevent the development of contractures and pressure sores, it is recommended that the patient be positioned appropriately in bed, rotated frequently (average 2 hours) and use an air mattress. The most basic approaches are to start passive, active-assistive, active range of motion (ROM), stretching exercises, preparation of resting splints, and teaching their use.

At least once a day during the flaccid period to maintain ROM, ROM 2–3 times a day after spasticity starts to develop exercises should be done. Bed if sitting balance is available exercises for sitting on the edge are given [23].

Despite significant advancements, individuals with spinal cord injury (SCI) continue to face a heightened risk of mortality, particularly in the initial stages following a traumatic event [15]. Furthermore, approximately 40% of patients require hospitalization within the first year post-SCI, a trend that persists over time, with urinary tract infections (UTIs), respiratory issues (including pneumonia), and skin complications such as pressure ulcers being the primary reasons for rehospitalization [24, 25]. Additionally, the socioeconomic impact of SCI is substantial, stemming from lost productivity alongside healthcare expenses. In the United States alone, annual direct hospitalization costs exceeded $2.2 billion in 2019, with indirect costs estimated at $77,334 per person [26].

Common complications following spinal cord injury (SCI) include pressure sores, pulmonary infections, urinary tract infections (UTIs), and venous thromboembolism (VTE), all of which pose significant risks to patient health [2, 27–29]. Pressure sores, characterized by localized injuries to the skin and underlying tissue, can escalate to serious infections and mortality if not properly addressed [30]. Pulmonary infections, often stemming from impaired cough and secretion clearance due to expiratory muscle dysfunction post-SCI, rank among the leading causes of mortality in these patients [2, 31].

UTIs can profoundly impact the daily activities and social functioning of individuals with SCI in the absence of effective management [32, 33]. The onset of VTE, encompassing deep vein thrombosis and pulmonary embolism, presents insidiously and poses a grave threat, contributing to elevated mortality rates among SCI patients [34]. Hence, the implementation of effective and standardized management protocols for these prevalent and detrimental complications is imperative for individuals with SCI.

The degree of respiratory system problems seen in patients with spinal cord injuries is related to the level and severity of the injury. Respiratory dysfunction is not expected in patients with lesions at or below the T12 level. In patients with lesions between T6 and T12, loss of function in abdominal and intercostal muscles may lead to difficulties in forceful expiration and coughing. Patients with lesions between T1 and T5 experience loss of function in intercostal muscles, resulting in severe problems with inspiratory and expiratory activities. In individuals with lower-level tetraplegia (C4–C8), there is no function in the intercostal and abdominal muscles, and expiratory power only occurs through the passive elasticity of the chest cage.

In patients with a last intact level at C3-4, accessory muscles can provide support to the acutely injured patient until they reach the emergency department, but respiratory failure is inevitable due to the inability of the diaphragm to generate sufficient contraction. In complete injuries at the C2 and above levels, mechanical ventilator support is required as the diaphragm and accessory muscles cannot function.

There are two important ways to prevent pulmonary complications in the early period: clearing secretions and ensuring the expansion of lung tissue. Assisted coughing, deep breathing and coughing, glossopharyngeal breathing, strengthening of respiratory muscles, and positioning are some of the approaches used in pulmonary rehabilitation for this purpose [35].

Patients with spinal cord injuries are at risk for deep vein thrombosis (DVT) and pulmonary embolism (PE) due to the combination of stasis, hypercoagulability, and intimal vascular damage known as Virchow's triad [36].

DVT prophylaxis should be initiated promptly after spinal cord injury. Mechanical prophylaxis in conjunction with anticoagulant therapy is recommended in all guidelines. Mechanical prophylaxis includes pneumatic compression, compression stockings, and bandaging with passive exercises. Anticoagulant prophylaxis should be initiated within the first 72 hours. Low molecular weight heparin (LMWH) has been found to be more effective and reliable compared to unfractionated heparin for anticoagulant prophylaxis [37].

According to the Spinal Cord Injury Guidelines Consortium, DVT prophylaxis is recommended until discharge in cases of motor incomplete injuries and for 8 weeks in uncomplicated complete injuries. For individuals with lower extremity fractures, prior thrombosis, cancer, heart failure, obesity, or age over 70 years with complete injuries, prophylaxis is recommended for 12 weeks [38].

4.2 Subacute period

During the transition from the intensive care unit to the rehabilitation unit/clinic, the goals are centered around restoring functionality. Activities on the mattress include turning, positioning on elbows and hands, short sitting, long sitting, and transfer training [39]. Using sliding boards to facilitate transfer is a fundamental step for transitioning to a wheelchair. Once the patient's sitting balance is established, ambulation with a wheelchair is taught. Patients with sensory impairment often should use an air mattress and perform push-ups at specific intervals (every 30 minutes, 15 seconds), which involves lifting the body with elbow extension [23].

The goal of balance and standing is initiated with the tilt-table period to stimulate necessary reflexes and regulate blood pressure (prevent orthostatic hypotension). In patients with upper thoracic lesions who tolerate the tilt-table period, verticalization exercises are introduced with a standing table. Parallel bar exercises are prioritized for walking initiation. Exercises at the parallel bars include standing up, maintaining balance, doing push-ups, turning while standing, advancing lower extremities with pelvic elevation, stepping, and practicing swing-through gait [39]. Device support may be necessary for ambulation; patients with complete thoracic injuries may require orthoses to support the knee and ankle. For patients performing only therapeutic ambulation, posterior-shell and dorsiflexor straps supporting the knee joint may be sufficient [23, 39, 40]. Although functional goals according to the level of injury are described in various sources (**Table 1**), achieved ambulation levels vary from person to person based on age, gender, upper extremity strength, body weight, patient motivation, and social support status [39].

4.3 Chronic period

The primary objective for both complete and incomplete paraplegic patients during the chronic phase is achieving independent mobilization. Ambulation serves various purposes including social interaction, domestic tasks, and exercise. For social ambulation, patients should be capable of walking unaided or with assistive devices for a distance of 50 meters. Domestic ambulation entails independent walking or requiring partial assistance, while exercise ambulation necessitates advanced assistance for walking or transferring. Ambulation potential is influenced by factors such as injury level, age, weight, general health status, motivation, and spasticity. Typically, patients with injuries at or above the T10 level can ambulate for exercise. Those with injuries ranging from T11 to L2 can manage domestic ambulation, while patients with more distal injuries can engage in social ambulation [40].

For patients who have completed the rehabilitation process, the necessary steps before discharge are summarized in **Table 2**. All devices for discharge should be

C2-3: Requires artificial respiration device, completely dependent on activities of daily living (ADL)
C4: Tongue, jaw, or pneumatically controlled motorized wheelchair, completely dependent on ADL
C5: Can perform ADL with special equipment, hand-controlled motorized wheelchair
C6: Grip achieved with tenodesis, joystick-controlled wheelchair, hand-controlled car
C7: Independent in transfers, except for ramp access, with standard wheelchair (WC)
C8-T1: Independent in ADL, WC mobility
T2-10: Standing with orthosis and therapeutic ambulation
T11-L2: Walking with long leg braces and crutches for household ambulation
L3-S3: Walking with short leg braces and forearm crutches for community ambulation.

Table 1.
Complete spinal cord injury level and targeted functional status [11].

Preparation of medication, supplies, devices, and rest report
Procurement of necessary devices and equipment
Provision of orthoses
Provision of medications
Supply of catheters
Home modifications
Scheduling follow-up appointments

Table 2.
Pre-discharge procedures [40].

prepared, catheters should be provided, and home modifications (such as toilet, bathroom handrails, widening doorways to accommodate wheelchair access, etc.) should be explained since the rehabilitation process will continue at home. Patients and their families should be informed about possible complications [23, 39]. Returning to work or gaining employment after spinal cord injury is among the most important indicators of community participation. This contributes to the individual's societal value and provides economic independence. According to a study conducted by Gündüz et al. in our country, the employment rate of individuals with spinal cord injury ranges from 14–36% [41]. Following discharge, patients diagnosed with spinal cord injury are recommended to be followed up by an experienced team; however, there are no guidelines regarding the content and frequency of these follow-ups. The first follow-up after discharge is recommended 3 months later, followed by every 3–6 months in the first 2 years depending on the patient's condition, and then annually for stable patients after 2 years [40]. Recommendations for the follow-up of individuals with spinal cord injury are reviewed below [42].

4.4 Transportation

Daily Follow-up Patients with SCI should perform daily skin checks for pressure ulcers.

Monthly Follow-up Individuals with SCI should perform monthly self-examinations; women should examine their breasts, and men should examine their testicles.

Annual Follow-up Both healthy individuals and those with SCI should undergo annual general health check-ups, fecal occult blood testing, mammography for women over 40 years of age, detailed eye examinations for those over 55 years of age, and prostate-specific antigen (PSA) testing and digital rectal examination for men over 75 years of age.

Individuals should undergo a complete blood count, biochemical tests, breast examinations for women, gynecological evaluations, and Pap smears at least every 2–3 years. In addition to these, individuals with SCI should have their weight and blood pressure checked regularly, and those with injuries at thoracic levels eight and above should receive flu vaccinations. Patients should undergo annual follow-ups in the first 5 years and then at least every 2–3 years, including medical history, complete physical examination (ISNCSCI assessment, joint range of motion, contractures, functional status, etc.), urological system assessment, posture, orthoses and devices, and full skin assessment.

4.5 5-year follow-up

For healthy individuals, lipid profiling after the age of 35, sigmoidoscopy, and CT colonography after the age of 50 are recommended. In individuals with SCI, in addition to these, respiratory function testing and a review of lifestyle changes are recommended.

4.6 10-year follow-up

For healthy individuals, tetanus vaccine boosters and colonoscopy are recommended. Additionally, pneumococcal vaccination is recommended for patients with injuries at thoracic levels eight and above.

5. Conclusion

Spinal cord injury (SCI) is a devastating condition, one of the most complex clinical situations a physician may encounter, affecting nearly all systems of the body. Ensuring psychological adaptation and providing rehabilitation that teaches daily life activities are essential for individuals with SCI to be productive members of society. Necessary adjustments should be made to facilitate patients' return to society, and the community should be educated about the primary prevention of SCI.

Author details

Zeynep Karakuzu Güngör
Batman Training and Research Hospital, Batman, Turkey

*Address all correspondence to: zeynepkarakuzu@hotmail.com.tr

References

[1] Mekki M, Delgado AD, Fry A, Putrino D, Huang V. Robotic rehabilitation and spinal cord injury: A narrative review. Neurotherapeutics. 2018;**15**(3):604-617

[2] Ahuja CS, Wilson JR, Nori S, Kotter MRN, Druschel C, Curt A, et al. Traumatic spinal cord injury. Nature Reviews Disease Primers. 2017;**3**:17018

[3] López-Dolado E. Nontraumatic myelopathies. Medicine-Programa de Formación Médica Continuada Acreditado. 2019;**12**(75):4401-4411

[4] Ding W, Hu S, Wang P, Kang H, Peng R, Dong Y, et al. Spinal cord injury: The global incidence, prevalence, and disability from the global burden of disease study 2019. Spine. 2022;**47**:1532-1540

[5] Ma X, Wang X, Ma X, Zhang X, Gong X, Sun R, et al. An update on the roles of circular RNAs in spinal cord injury. Molecular Neurobiology. 2022;**59**:2620-2628

[6] Golestani A, Shobeiri P, Sadeghi-Naini M, Jazayeri SB, Maroufi SF, Ghodsi Z, et al. Epidemiology of traumatic spinal cord injury in developing countries from 2009 to 2020: A systematic review and meta-analysis. Neuroepidemiology. 2022;**56**:219-239

[7] Nistor-Cseppento CD, Gherle A, Negrut N, Bungau SG, Sabau AM, Radu AF, et al. The Outcomes of Robotic Rehabilitation Assisted Devices Following Spinal Cord Injury and the Prevention of Secondary Associated Complications. Vol. 58. Medicina. Kaunas, Lithuania: Nobel Tıp Kitabevleri; 2022. p. 1447

[8] Khandelwal A, Shafer LA, Ethans K. Does severity of spinal cord injury predict likelihood of suffering chronically from severe depression and anxiety? Spinal Cord Series and Cases. 2022;**8**:58

[9] Rathnayake L, Baminiwatta A, Chandradasa M, Fernando L. Depressive morbidity among persons with spinal cord injury in Sri Lanka and the diagnostic utility of the Centre for Epidemiologic Studies Depression Scale. Asian Journal of Psychiatry. 2022;**69**:103006

[10] Singh V, Mitra S. Psychophysiological impact of spinal cord injury: Depression, coping and heart rate variability. The Journal of Spinal Cord Medicine. 2022;**12**(3):1-9. (Online ahead of print)

[11] Malekzadeh H, Golpayegani M, Ghodsi Z, Sadeghi-Naini M, Asgardoon M, Baigi V, et al. Direct cost of illness for spinal cord injury: A systematic review. Global Spine Journal. 2022;**12**:1267-1281

[12] Alizadeh A, Dyck SM, Karimi-Abdolrezaee S. Traumatic spinal cord injury: An overview of pathophysiology, models and acute injury mechanisms. Frontiers in Neurology. 2019;**10**:282

[13] Chiu WT, Lin HC, Lam C, Chu SF, Chiang YH, Tsai SH. Review paper: Epidemiology of traumatic spinal cord injury: Comparisons between developed and developing countries. Asia-Pacific Journal of Public Health. 2010;**22**(1):9-18

[14] Golestani A, Shobeiri P, Sadeghi-Naini M, Jazayeri SB, Marouf SF, Ghodsi Z, et al. Epidemiology of traumatic spinal cord injury in developing countries from 2009 to 2020:

A systematic review and meta-analysis. Neuroepidemiology. 2022;**56**(4):219-239

[15] Selassie AW, Varma A, Saunders LL, Welldaregay W. Determinants of inhospital death after acute spinal cord injury: A population-based study. Spinal Cord. 2013;**51**(1):48-54

[16] Bryce T. Spinal cord injury. In: Cifu DX, editor. Braddom's Physical Medicine and Rehabilitation. 5th ed. Philadelphia: Saunders; 2016. pp. 1095-1136

[17] Kirshblum SC, Biering-Sorensen F, Betz R, Burns S, Donovan W, Graves DE, et al. International standards for neurological classification of spinal cord injury: Cases with classification challenges. The Journal of Spinal Cord Medicine. 2014;**37**(2):120-127

[18] Kirshblum SC, Waring W, Biering-Sorensen F, Burns SP, Johansen M, Schmidt-Read M, et al. Reference for the 2011 revision of the international standards for neurological classification of spinal cord injury. The Journal of Spinal Cord Medicine. 2011;**34**(6):547-554

[19] Anjum A, Yazid MD, Daud MF, Idris J, Hwei Ng AM, Naicker AS, et al. Spinal cord injury: Pathophysiology, multimolecular interactions, and underlying recovery mechanisms. International Journal of Molecular Sciences. 2020;**21**(20):7533

[20] Dumont RJ, Okonkwo DO, Verma S, Hurlbert RJ, Boulos PT, Ellegala DB, et al. Acute spinal cord injury, part I: Pathophysiologic mechanisms. Clinical Neuropharmacology. 2001;**24**(5):254-264

[21] Ditunno JF, Little JW, Tessler A, Burns AS. Spinal shock revisited: A fourphase model. Spinal Cord. 2004;**42**(7):383-395

[22] Kesani AK, Urquhart JC, Bedard N, Leelapattana P, Siddiqi F, Gurr KR, et al. Systemic Inflammatory Response Syndrome in Patients with Spinal Cord Injury: Does its Presence at Admission Affect Patient Outcomes? Philadelphia: Elsevier; 2016

[23] Bryce TN, Ragnarrson KT, Stein AB, Sorenson FB. Spinal cord injury. In: Braddom RL, editor. Physical Medicine and Rehabilitation. Philadelphia: Saunders, Clinical article. J Neurosurg Spine. 2011;21(2):296-302. 2011:1293-1346

[24] Krause JS, Saunders LL. Risk of hospitalizations after spinal cord injury: Relationship with biographic, injury, educational, and behavioral factors. Spinal Cord. 2009;**47**(9):692-697

[25] Cardenas DD, Hofman JM, Kirshblum S, McKinley W. Etiology and incidence of rehospitalization after traumatic spinal cord injury: A mul-ticenter analysis. Archives of Physical Medicine and Rehabilitation. 2004;**85**(11):1757-1763

[26] Lo J, Chan L, Flynn S. A systematic review of the incidence, prevalence, costs, and activity/work limitations of amputation, osteoarthritis, rheu-matoid arthritis, back pain, multiple sclerosis, spinal cord injury, stroke, and traumatic brain injury in the United States: A 2019 update. Archives of Physical Medicine and Rehabilitation. 2021;**102**(1):115-131

[27] Yuan S, Shi Z, Cao F, Li J, Feng S. Epidemiological features of spinal cord injury in China: A systematic review. Frontiers in Neurology. 2018;**9**:683

[28] Grossman RG, Frankowski RF, Burau KD, Toups EG, Crommett JW, Johnson MM, et al. Incidence and severity of acute complications

after spinal cord injury. Journal of Neurosurgery. Spine. 2012;**171 Suppl**:119-128

[29] Aito S. Complications during the acute phase of traumatic spinal cord lesions. Spinal Cord. 2003;**41**(11):629-635

[30] Edsberg LE, Black JM, Goldberg M, McNichol L, Moore L, Sieggreen M. Revised national pressure ulcer advisory panel pressure injury staging system: Revised pressure injury staging system. Journal of Wound, Ostomy, and Continence Nursing. 2020;**20**:335-350

[31] Brown R, DiMarco AF, Hoit JD, Garshick E. Respiratory dysfunction and management in spinal cord injury. Respiratory Care. 2006;**51**(8):853-868. discussion 69-70

[32] Pannek J. Treatment of urinary tract infection in persons with spinal cord injury: Guidelines, evidence, and clinical practice. A questionnaire based survey and review of the literature. The Journal of Spinal Cord Medicine. 2011;**34**(1):11-15

[33] Everaert K, Lumen N, Kerckhaert W, Willaert P, van Driel M. Urinary tract infections in spinal cord injury: Prevention and treatment guidelines. Acta Clinica Belgica. 2009;**64**(4):335-340

[34] Anderson FA Jr, Spencer FA. Risk factors for venous thromboembolism. Circulation. 2003;**107**(23 Suppl. 1):I9-I16

[35] Grimm DR, Schilero GJ, Spungen AM, Bauman WA, Lesser M. Salmeterol improves pulmonary function in persons with tetraplegia. Lung. 2006;**184**(6):335-339

[36] Green D, Sullivan S, Simpson J, Soltysik RC, Yarnold PR. Evolving risk for thromboembolism in spinal cord injury (SPIRATE study). American Journal of Physical Medicine & Rehabilitation. 2005;**84**(6):420-422

[37] Teasell RW, Hsieh JT, Aubut JA, Eng JJ, Krassioukov A, Tu L. Spinal cord Injury rehabilitation evidence review research team: Venous thromboembolism after spinal cord injury. Archives of Physical Medicine and Rehabilitation. 2009;**90**(2):232-245

[38] Prevention of Thromboembolism in Spinal Cord Injury. Consortium for spinal cord medicine. The Journal of Spinal Cord Medicine. 1997;**20**:259-283

[39] Güzel R, Uysal FG. Spinal kord yaralanmaları. In: Dursun OHE, Dursun N, editors. Tıbbi Rehabilitasyon. İstanbul: Nobel Tıp Kitabevleri; 2004. pp. 627-645

[40] Alaca R. Spinal kord yaralanmasında rehabilitasyon. In: Beyazova M, Kutsal YG, editors. Fiziksel Tıp ve Rehabilitasyon. Ankara: Güneş Tıp Kitabevleri; 2011. pp. 2893-2916

[41] Gunduz B, Erhan B, Bardak AN. Employment among spinal cord injured patients living in Turkey: A cross-sectional study. IJRR. 2010;**33**(3):275-278

[42] Erhan B. Medulla spinalis yaralanmalı hastalarda geç dönem takip protokolü. Turkish Journal of Physical Medicine and Rehabilitation. 2006;**52**(Suppl. B):818-820